Real Food, Happy Gut

A Gut Health Cookbook for People Who Hate Supplements

Clyde Owen Leonard

This book is for general informational and educational purposes only and is not intended to serve as professional medical advice, diagnosis, or treatment. Readers should consult with a qualified healthcare provider before making significant dietary changes, starting a new health protocol, or if they have specific medical conditions or concerns.

The publisher and author make no guarantees regarding specific health outcomes, digestive improvements, or physical results from applying the methods in this book. Every individual's biological response to dietary changes is unique, and readers assume full personal responsibility for their choices and actions.

Any names, characters, examples, and scenarios depicted in this book are used for illustrative purposes only. They are entirely fictional or heavily modified to protect privacy, and they are not intended to harm, misrepresent, or identify any actual person, living or dead, or any specific entity.

First Edition:2026

ISBN: 979-8-90599-196-7

Table of Contents

The $50 Billion Supplement Lie

You know that feeling when you stand in front of your kitchen cabinet at seven o'clock in the morning, staring at a row of plastic bottles? There is the daily probiotic that cost forty dollars and needs to stay in the fridge. Next to it is the big tub of swamp-green powder your coworker swore would fix your bloating. Then there is the bottle of digestive enzymes, the magnesium capsules, and maybe a jar of fiber gummies just for good measure. You scoop the green dust into a shaker bottle, add water, and shake it up. You unscrew the lid, smell that grassy, chalky odor, and hold your breath while you swallow it down.

It tastes awful. It costs a fortune. And truth is, your stomach still feels like a blown-up balloon by three o'clock in the afternoon.

If this sounds like your morning routine, I need you to hear something right now. You are not failing at health. You are not doing it wrong because you missed a dose of your greens powder or because you bought the thirty-billion colony probiotic instead of the fifty-billion one. You have been sold a bill of goods by a wellness industry that cares a whole lot more about recurring monthly subscriptions than about your digestive tract.

Look, we need to be honest about how we got here. We live in a fast-paced, high-stress culture where eating sit-down meals made from scratch feels like a luxury from a bygone era. When your stomach hurts, when you feel sluggish, and when your jeans don't zip comfortably anymore, it is completely natural to look for a quick solution. The supplement brands know this. They spend millions of dollars every year on sleek packaging and social media ads designed to make you feel like your body is broken and their proprietary blend is the only magic wrench that can fix it.

But here is the catch. You cannot buy a healthy gut in a plastic tub. You have to cook it. And I am going to show you exactly why ordinary grocery store food works better than any pill you will ever swallow.

How The Wellness Industry Trapped Us

Let's talk about the sheer size of the supplement business. Right now, dietary supplements represent a global industry worth over fifty billion dollars, and it grows bigger every single year. Walk into any pharmacy or grocery store, and you will see entire aisles dedicated to digestion. There are pills promising to balance your flora, powders claiming to reset your system, and teas that guarantee a flat stomach by tomorrow morning.

Why do we buy this stuff? Because we are exhausted. We are working longer hours, managing stressful family lives, and trying to survive on coffee and quick sandwiches eaten over our keyboards. When an advertisement pops up on your phone promising that one scoop of green powder a day will replace thirty vegetables, fix your digestion, and give you boundless energy, you want to believe it. I get it. It sounds like a lifeline when you are drowning in fatigue and stomach cramps.

The problem is that the marketing rarely matches the medical reality. Most commercial supplements are sold without strict clinical testing to prove they actually do what the label claims. When researchers test commercial probiotic capsules off retail shelves, they frequently find that the live bacteria inside have already died from heat exposure during shipping or warehouse storage. Even if the bacteria are still alive when you swallow the capsule, a huge number of them get completely destroyed by your harsh stomach acid before they ever reach your lower intestines where they belong.

When major medical bodies have reviewed the evidence, they have concluded that most dietary supplements marketed for digestion lack robust clinical proof that they improve gut health or change long-term outcomes in otherwise healthy people (Su et al., 2020).

That quote right there tells you what doctors and researchers have known for years. We are throwing hard-earned money at products that mostly give us very expensive urine and a false sense of security. It is time to stop blaming your body and start looking at the real science of how human digestion actually works.

The Mystery Of The Food Matrix

To understand why ordinary food beats expensive pills every single time, we need to talk about a scientific concept called the *food matrix*. Don't worry, we are not getting into advanced chemistry here. The food matrix is just a fancy way of describing how all the different parts of a whole food are physically and biologically packaged together by nature.

When you eat a whole apple, you are not just taking a dose of Vitamin C. You are eating water, soluble fiber, insoluble fiber, natural sugars, minerals, and plant compounds called polyphenols. All of those ingredients are locked together in a specific physical structure. When you chew that apple and swallow it, your body has to work to break that structure apart. That work slows down digestion, keeps your blood sugar steady, and carries nutrients safely through your acidic stomach all the way down to your colon. Once those nutrients reach the colon, they act as the exact fuel your good bacteria need to thrive.

Now, compare that apple to a synthetic Vitamin C pill or a scoop of isolated fiber powder. In a factory, chemists strip away the surrounding nutrients, remove the natural water, and crush the remaining chemicals into a fine dust. When you swallow that powder, there is no physical structure left to slow things down. There is no biological teamwork happening between different nutrients. Your body absorbs a big spike of the chemical right away in the upper stomach, and very little of it ever makes it down to the lower gut to feed your microbiome.

Researchers call this natural teamwork food cooperation. When vitamins, minerals, and fibers travel together inside real food, they protect each other and help your body absorb what it needs at the right pace.

Nutrition researchers call this food synergy: the nutrients in a whole food work together in ways that isolated supplements simply cannot reproduce (Jacobs & Tapsell, 2013).

Think of your digestive system like a wood-burning stove. Whole foods are like solid, dry oak logs. You put them in the stove, they catch fire slowly, and they burn steadily for hours, giving off consistent heat without burning the house down. Supplements are like throwing a bucket of gasoline into that same stove. You get an instant, blinding flash of heat and smoke, and then two seconds later, the fire is completely out and you are left in the cold. Why keep paying top dollar for gasoline when you can get a cord of firewood at the local market for a fraction of the price?

Buying Gut Health Versus Cooking It

Let's get down to brass tacks and talk about your wallet. The financial toll of what I call pill fatigue is staggering, especially when you add it up over a full year. Most health-conscious people don't just buy one product. They get caught in a cycle of buying a base green powder, a daily probiotic, a prebiotic fiber supplement, and maybe a specialty tea or gummy.

To see how this plays out in real life, let's look at Sarah. Sarah is a thirty-eight-year-old accountant living in Ohio. For two years, she struggled with daily bloating, afternoon brain fog, and unpredictable bowel habits. She went to her doctor, who told her she had mild digestive sensitivity and suggested she eat more fiber. But Sarah was busy during tax season, so she went online instead. She started watching wellness videos and soon found herself subscribed to a monthly delivery of a premium greens powder that cost eighty-five dollars a bottle. Then she added a refrigerated daily probiotic for forty dollars a month, and a specialized digestive enzyme complex for another thirty-five dollars.

Every morning, Sarah spent ten minutes mixing powders and swallowing capsules. She spent one hundred and sixty dollars every single month—nearly two thousand dollars a year—just trying to make her stomach stop hurting. And you know what happened? Her bloating actually got worse. Why? Because the synthetic alcohols and flavorings in the green powder were irritating her stomach lining, while her actual diet still consisted of toasted bagels, takeout sandwiches, and processed dinner kits that starved her lower gut bacteria.

When Sarah finally sat down and looked at her bank statements, she was furious. She stopped her auto-ship subscriptions that very afternoon. Instead of spending forty dollars a week on bottles and tubs, she took twenty dollars to her local supermarket. She bought a giant bag of steel-cut oats, a sack of dried brown lentils, three heads of cabbage, a bag of carrots, and a bunch of bananas.

Within two weeks of switching to real, simple grocery store foods, Sarah's bloating went down by half. She wasn't gagging down green swamp water anymore. She was eating warm oatmeal topped with mashed bananas in the morning, and comforting lentil soup with sweet carrots for lunch. Her digestion became regular for the first time in years, her afternoon brain fog lifted, and she put fourteen hundred dollars back into her savings account over the next ten months.

You do not need an accountant's salary to afford a healthy microbiome. In fact, some of the absolute best foods for your digestive tract are the cheapest items sitting on the bottom shelves of your local grocery store. A fifty-cent can of black beans or a two-dollar head of green cabbage contains more genuine gut-healing power than a hundred-dollar jar of designer wellness powder ever could.

My Promise to You

I want to be very clear about what this book is and what it is definitely not.

This is not a restrictive diet book that is going to tell you to stop eating every food you love. You are not going to see any instructions telling you to drink lemon water for three days to cleanse your system. Your liver and your kidneys already do a fantastic job of cleaning your blood every second of the day, and they do it for free. We are not doing cleanses here, and we are certainly not going to count every single calorie or weigh every grain of rice on a tiny digital scale.

This is a cookbook and a practical road map for people who want to feel good in their bodies without turning their kitchens into a chemistry lab. My promise to you is simple. Inside these pages, you are going to find eighty-five delicious, easy-to-cook recipes that use ordinary whole foods you can buy at any neighborhood supermarket. You will not find a single recipe that asks you to buy an expensive supplement powder, a specialty capsule, or an obscure herb ordered from across the globe.

We are going to use real food—hearty stews, comforting grain bowls, roasted vegetables, simple soups, and yes, even desserts—to feed the good bacteria in your stomach so they can do their job properly. We will use plain talk, easy steps, and flavor-packed ingredients to get your digestion working smoothly again. No magic tricks. No overpriced pills. Just good food and solid science.

How To Use This Book

To get the most out of this book, you want to approach it like a practical tool rather than a textbook you have to read from cover to cover in one sitting. I have organized the chapters to walk you through a logical sequence that builds your confidence both in your body and in your kitchen.

First, we are going to look at the basic mechanics of your digestive system in plain, everyday language. You need to understand who the players are inside your stomach so you know why you are feeding them certain foods. Once we get the science out of the way without any confusing medical jargon, we will move straight into your kitchen. We will talk about how to set up your pantry without spending a fortune, how to read grocery labels without getting tricked by clever marketing, and how to prep food so cooking dinner on a busy Tuesday night feels effortless.

After your kitchen is ready, we jump into the recipes. I have grouped them by meals and daily needs so you can easily grab what fits your schedule. Whether you need a quick five-minute breakfast before rushing out the door, a packable lunch that won't make you want to nap at your desk, or a hearty dinner that your entire family will actually enjoy eating with you, you will find it here. Later in the book, we will cover what to do when things go wrong—how to handle a sudden stomach upset, what to order when you are dining out at a restaurant, and how to track your progress without spending hundreds of dollars on medical testing kits.

Take it one chapter at a time, one meal at a time. If you mess up a recipe or eat a greasy fast-food burger on a Friday night, don't sweat it. Your gut bacteria are remarkably resilient. They don't demand perfection; they just want consistency over the long haul.

Action Step The Supplement Audit

Before we dive into how your microbiome actually works in the next chapter, we need to clear the slate. I want you to take fifteen minutes today to do a complete inventory of what you are putting into your body and what you are spending your money on. We call this the Supplement Audit.

Go to your kitchen cabinets, your pantry, your bathroom drawers, and anywhere else you stash health products. Pull out every single bottle, tub, dropper, and packet of supplements you currently own. Put them all on your kitchen table. Now, grab a pen and a piece of paper, or open the notes app on your phone. You are going to make a simple chart to see the reality of your current routine.

The Supplement Audit Worksheet

Take an honest look at the supplements you're currently using. The goal isn't to judge your choices—it's to understand what you're taking, why you're taking it, what it costs, and whether you've noticed any real benefits.

Supplement 1

Product Name: ____

Why did you buy it?

____

How often do you take it?

____

Monthly cost: $____________________

Have you noticed any real benefit?

____

____

Supplement 2

Product Name: ____

Why did you buy it?

____

How often do you take it?

____

Monthly cost: $____________________

Have you noticed any real benefit?

Supplement 3

Product Name: ______________________________

Why did you buy it?

How often do you take it?

Monthly cost: $__________________

Have you noticed any real benefit?

Your Totals

Total Monthly Spend: $__________________

Estimated Yearly Spend (Monthly × 12): $__________________

Be totally honest when you fill out the benefit line. If a forty-dollar bottle of pills has not clearly and noticeably improved your digestion, your energy, or your sleep after thirty days of consistent use, write down the word "None."

Once you add up that total monthly and yearly cost, take a good, hard look at that number. Imagine what you could do with that money if you weren't flushing it down the toilet on products that don't deliver. You are going to take a big chunk of that budget and redirect it toward delicious, fresh, high-quality groceries that will actually heal your system from the inside out. Put those bottles back in the cupboard for now, take a deep breath, and let's go meet the trillions of microscopic workers who are waiting to help you.

What We Covered Here

- **The wellness industry thrives on pill fatigue:** Companies spend billions selling isolated powders and capsules that often fail to survive stomach acid or deliver real medical benefits.
- **Whole foods have a built-in advantage:** The natural *food matrix* locks vitamins, minerals, and fibers together, allowing your body to absorb nutrients steadily and carry good bacteria safely to your lower gut.
- **You cannot buy gut health in a bottle:** Spending hundreds of dollars a month on supplements is usually a waste of money compared to spending twenty dollars on cheap, nutrient-dense grocery staples like beans, cabbage, and oats.
- **Consistency beats perfection:** You don't need extreme cleanses, complicated dieting rules, or expensive testing kits to heal your digestive tract; you just need simple, repeatable daily cooking habits.
- **Your kitchen is your best pharmacy:** By cutting out ineffective supplement subscriptions, you can save thousands of dollars a year while eating flavorful, satisfying meals that naturally solve bloating and fatigue.

Before We Move On

Take a second to congratulate yourself for taking a rational, hard look at your daily routine. It is not easy to admit when we have been spending good money on health products that don't actually work, but doing that honest assessment is the only way to break free from the marketing trap. Now that you know why isolated powders fall short of real food, you are ready to look under the hood of your digestive system. In the next chapter, we are going to walk through exactly how your gut microbiome operates without using a single piece of confusing medical jargon. You are going to learn why your stomach sometimes feels like it has a mind of its own, and how you can become the boss of your internal garden starting tonight. Ready? Let's turn the page.

Chapter 1: Meet Your Microbiome

(No PhD Required)

Let's clear the air right away. Whenever people start talking about gut health, the conversation usually turns into a science lecture full of big, intimidating words that sound like they belong in a medical school textbook. You hear people throwing around terms like *microbiota*, *short-chain fatty acids*, *lipopolysaccharides*, and *epithelial permeability*. By the time someone finishes explaining how it all works, your eyes have glazed over and you are ready to order a pizza just to stop thinking about it.

Here is the plain truth. You do not need a medical degree to understand how your digestion works, and you certainly don't need to memorize the Latin names of microscopic bacteria to stop your stomach from hurting. What you need is a simple, common-sense picture of what is actually happening inside your body after you swallow your food.

Once you see how the system is set up, all those confusing dietary rules you see on social media start to fall apart. You stop wondering whether you should buy this expensive pill or try that restrictive diet, because you finally understand what the little workers inside your belly actually need to do their jobs. So let's drop the medical jargon and talk about your digestive tract like normal human beings.

Your Internal Garden

Imagine that your digestive tract, specifically your large intestine, is a bustling, crowded community garden sitting right in the middle of your body. Scientists call this garden your *microbiome*. Inside this garden, there are trillions of tiny living microorganisms—mostly bacteria, along with some friendly yeasts and other microscopic helpers.

To give you an idea of just how crowded this garden is, consider this. There are roughly thirty-eight trillion microbial cells living inside your lower gut right now. That means you actually have more bacterial cells living inside your body than you have human cells making up your blood, your bones, and your muscles combined!

The most careful modern estimates put the number of bacteria in a seventy-kilogram adult at roughly thirty-eight trillion, about the same as, or slightly more than, the body's own thirty trillion human cells (Sender et al., 2016).

I know that idea can sound a little weird or even creepy at first. We grow up being told that bacteria are germs that cause diseases, and that we need to kill them with antibacterial soap and antibiotics. But the bacteria living in your gut garden are not invaders trying to make you sick. They are your dedicated workforce. They are like a massive crew of master gardeners who work twenty-four hours a day, seven days a week, keeping you healthy from the inside out.

When your internal garden is thriving, these worker bugs perform all sorts of amazing tasks for you. They break down tough food pieces that your stomach couldn't digest on its own. They manufacture vital nutrients, including Vitamin K and several B vitamins, right there on the spot. They build a thick, protective wall along your intestinal lining to keep toxins and bad germs from leaking into your bloodstream. They even act as drill sergeants for your immune system, teaching your infection-fighting cells the difference between friendly food and dangerous invaders.

Now, what happens if that garden gets ignored? If you stop feeding your good workers and let the soil go dry, weeds start to take over. In your gut, those weeds are the troublesome, inflammation-causing bacteria that love sugar and refined flour. When the weeds crowd out the helpful master gardeners, your protective intestinal wall gets thin and leaky. You start experiencing gas, painful bloating, unpredictable trips to the bathroom, and a general feeling of sluggishness. The secret to fixing those symptoms isn't to dump expensive chemical bug sprays into the garden. The secret is simply to nourish the good soil and feed your helpful workers so they can crowd those troublesome weeds right out of the patch.

Seeds Versus Fertilizer

If you have spent any time looking at health articles or shopping in a supplement aisle, you have probably bumped into two words that sound almost identical: *probiotics* and *prebiotics*. Because they sound so much alike, supplement brands often blur them together to sell you expensive package deals. But understanding the difference between these two things is the single most important lesson you will ever learn about your digestion. Let's break them down using our garden story.

A *probiotic* is simply a live, friendly bacterial seed. When you eat a food or swallow a pill containing probiotics, you are dropping new bacterial seeds into your digestive garden, hoping they will take root and grow alongside the workers who are already living there. You can find these live seeds in naturally fermented foods like yogurt, kefir, traditional sauerkraut, kimchi, and aged cheeses.

A *prebiotic*, on the other hand, is not a living bug at all. A prebiotic is the fertilizer and soil food that feeds the bugs already living in your system. In practical terms, prebiotics are specific types of dietary fiber and natural plant compounds found in everyday foods like garlic, onions, oats, apples, beans, asparagus, and bananas. Your human stomach cannot digest these fibrous plant fibers on its own. They pass through your upper stomach untouched and land safely in your lower intestine, where your bacterial workers eagerly chew them up for dinner.

When your good bacteria eat that prebiotic plant fiber, something wonderful happens. As they digest the fiber, they produce magical little health molecules called *short-chain fatty acids*. Think of these molecules as the golden harvest of your garden. These helpful fatty acids immediately go to work reducing inflammation in your gut lining, signaling your brain that you are full and satisfied, and giving your body a clean, steady source of daily energy.

Dietary fiber is the main fuel your colon bacteria ferment, and that fermentation produces short-chain fatty acids that help keep the gut lining and your metabolism in balance (Makki et al., 2018).

Now, let's look at why swallowing expensive probiotic pills often fails. Imagine you go to a hardware store and spend a hundred dollars on a bag of fancy grass seed. You take that seed home and throw it onto a dry, cracked, weed-choked dirt patch in your backyard. Then you walk inside, refuse to water it, and refuse to put down any fertilizer or topsoil. Are you going to get a lush, green lawn? Of course not! Those expensive seeds will just blow away in the wind or die on the hard dirt.

That is exactly what happens when you swallow a forty-dollar probiotic capsule while eating a diet of processed fast food, white bread, and sugary snacks. You are dropping live seeds onto a barren, unfertilized patch of dirt inside your gut. Without prebiotic fiber—the fertilizer—to feed them, those newly swallowed bacteria starve to death within a day or two and pass right out of your system without doing a bit of good. If you want a healthy microbiome, you must stop obsessing over buying fancy seeds and start focusing on feeding the soil with simple, fibrous plant fertilizer.

The Thirty Plants A Week Rule

So, if feeding the soil with plant fertilizer is the key to a happy gut, how do you actually do it in the real world without carrying a scientific nutrition chart around with you? A few years ago, a group of scientists ran a massive research study called the American Gut Project. They collected and analyzed gut bacteria samples from over ten thousand people all around the world to see what the healthiest, happiest digestive systems had in common.

The researchers expected to find that people on strict specialty diets—like low-carb, low-fat, or pure vegan diets—would have the best microbiomes. But that wasn't what they found at all. The single biggest factor that predicted a strong, healthy, diverse gut garden wasn't what foods people excluded from their plates. It was the sheer variety of different plants they ate over the course of a normal week.

Specifically, the researchers discovered that people who ate thirty or more different plant types every week had vastly more diverse and resilient gut bacteria than people who ate ten or fewer plant types a week.

In the American Gut Project, people who ate more than thirty different types of plants each week had noticeably more diverse gut bacteria than those who ate ten or fewer (McDonald et al., 2018).

Why does variety matter so much? Because your trillions of gut workers are not picky eaters who all like the same dish. Your garden contains hundreds of different bacterial families, and each family has its own favorite food. One family of good bugs might thrive on the specific soluble fiber found in oatmeal. Another family might prefer the tough skins of red beans. Yet another family loves the colorful antioxidants found in blueberries, while a fourth family goes crazy for the pungent sulfur compounds in crushed garlic.

If you eat the exact same breakfast, lunch, and dinner every single day—even if it is a healthy meal like chicken breast, brown rice, and broccoli—you are only feeding two or three families of bacteria. The rest of your helpful workers, starving for their own favorite foods, slowly die off from neglect. When you lose those workers, you lose the specific health benefits they provide, and your garden becomes weak and easily overrun by weeds.

Now, before you panic and think that eating thirty different plants a week sounds like an impossible full-time job, let me put your mind at ease. When we say "plants," we are not just talking about big bowls of leafy green salad or boiled vegetables. In the world of gut science, a plant is any whole food that grows out of the ground. That means every single one of the following categories counts toward your weekly score:

- **Fruits:** Apples, bananas, berries, oranges, peaches, avocados, and tomatoes.
- **Vegetables:** Onions, carrots, spinach, cabbage, peppers, broccoli, and sweet potatoes.
- **Whole Grains:** Rolled oats, brown rice, quinoa, barley, whole wheat, and buckwheat.
- **Legumes:** Black beans, chickpeas, brown lentils, kidney beans, and green peas.
- **Nuts and Seeds:** Walnuts, almonds, chia seeds, flaxseeds, sunflower seeds, and pumpkin seeds.
- **Herbs and Spices:** Cinnamon, garlic powder, dried oregano, fresh basil, ginger, black pepper, and turmeric.

When you count spices, seeds, and grains alongside your normal fruits and vegetables, hitting thirty different plants a week is surprisingly simple. A morning bowl of oatmeal cooked with a diced apple, a sprinkle of cinnamon, a spoonful of chia seeds, and a handful of walnuts gives you five different plants before eight o'clock in the morning! Add a little garlic and onion to your evening soup, and toss in some carrots and lentils, and you are already halfway to your weekly goal without ever eating a sad desk salad.

Why Your Stomach Controls Your Mood

Have you ever had a sudden feeling of intense nervousness right before a job interview and felt your stomach do a literal flip-flop? Or maybe you received some bad news and instantly felt sick to your stomach, like you couldn't eat a bite of food if your life depended on it? We use everyday expressions like having "butterflies in your stomach" or making a "gut decision" all the time. Turns out, those phrases are not just poetic figures of speech. They describe a real, physical communication highway running straight through your body.

Scientists call this connection the *gut-brain axis*. You actually have a massive network of over one hundred million nerve cells embedded right inside the walls of your digestive tract. This network is so large and complex that researchers frequently refer to it as your "second brain." Connecting your main brain in your head to this second brain in your belly is a thick, winding nerve bundle called the *vagus nerve*.

Think of the vagus nerve like a high-speed, two-way telephone line operating twenty-four hours a day. Your brain uses this line to send messages down to your stomach, telling it when to release digestive juices or when to speed up muscle contractions. But here is the amazing part: your gut sends roughly nine times more messages up to your head than your head sends down to your gut! Your digestive tract is constantly reporting back to your central nervous system, telling it how safe, fed, and relaxed your body feels.

This communication line explains why poor gut health takes such a heavy toll on your emotions and mental well-being. Consider the story of serotonin. Serotonin is often called the "happiness chemical" because it regulates your mood, your sleep quality, and your general feelings of calmness and well-being. Most people assume that serotonin is made entirely inside your brain. But medical research shows that roughly ninety percent of your body's total serotonin is actually produced down in your digestive tract by your specialized gut cells and bacterial workers!

Most of the body's serotonin, well over ninety percent, is made not in the brain but by specialized enterochromaffin cells in the gut, and the gut's bacteria help drive that production (Yano et al., 2015).

When your internal garden is full of weeds—when you are bloated, inflamed, and feeding your system a steady stream of highly refined junk food—your good bacteria cannot help produce that vital serotonin. Instead, the inflammation in your gut lining sends a steady stream of distress signals up the vagus nerve telephone line right into your brain. Your central nervous system receives those alarm bells and triggers your stress hormones.

The result? You wake up at three o'clock in the morning with your heart racing in a worry spiral, or you feel a persistent, low-grade anxiety all day long that you just can't shake. You might think you are losing your mind or that you need to try advanced mental relaxation techniques, when the root cause of your nervous tension is actually sitting right there in your inflamed lower intestines.

This connection is a two-way street, which means we have to be smart about how we treat our bodies. When you are constantly stressed out by work or family pressures, your brain sends panic signals down the vagus nerve that actually shut down your digestion, reduce your protective stomach acids, and starve your good bacteria. And when your digestion breaks down, your gut sends distress signals right back up to keep your brain in a state of alarm.

To break that exhausting loop, you don't need magic pills. You just need to start feeding your belly calming, anti-inflammatory whole foods that help your good bacteria produce serotonin again. When your belly feels peaceful, fed, and nourished, it calls up your brain on that vagus nerve telephone line and says, "Everything is fine down here. You can relax now."

The Hunter Gatherer Versus The Modern Eater

To see how drastically our modern lifestyle has impacted our internal garden, let's look at a fascinating real-world scientific comparison. For years, medical researchers have traveled to Tanzania in East Africa to study a traditional group of people called the Hadza. The Hadza are among the very last true hunter-gatherer tribes left on planet Earth. They live off the land just like our human ancestors did thousands of years ago, hunting wild game and gathering wild berries, tubers, baobab fruit, and honey.

When scientists examined the gut microbiome of Hadza tribespeople, they were absolutely stunned by what they found under the microscope. The Hadza possess the most diverse, resilient, and robust gut bacterial communities ever recorded in human history. Their internal gardens are overflowing with helpful bug families that have completely disappeared from the digestive tracts of average people living in modern Western countries. They rarely suffer from common digestive complaints like chronic constipation, irritable bowel syndrome, or inflammatory autoimmune disorders.

Studies of the Hadza, a hunter-gatherer community in Tanzania, show a remarkably diverse gut microbiome that even shifts with the seasons, diversity that is largely missing in industrialized Western populations (Smits et al., 2017).

Now, why is their gut health so bulletproof compared to ours? Let's put a Hadza tribesman side by side with a fictional modern desk worker to see the contrast. Let's call our modern worker Mark. Mark is a forty-two-year-old project manager living in Chicago. He is a nice guy, he works hard, and he tries his best to take care of his family. But let's look at a typical Tuesday in Mark's life compared to the Hadza reality.

When Mark wakes up, he grabs a sweet coffee drink and a toasted white flour bagel on his way to the office. For lunch, he eats a turkey sandwich made with refined bread and a bag of potato chips while answering emails at his desk. For dinner, he is too exhausted to cook, so he orders a pepperoni pizza and drinks a couple of sodas. Across that entire day, Mark consumed roughly eight to ten grams of dietary fiber, and he ate maybe three or four different plant types—mostly wheat flour, processed potatoes, and whatever tomato paste was smeared on the pizza. His digestive system got almost no prebiotic fertilizer, and his helpful bacterial workers spent the day starving.

Meanwhile, over in Tanzania, our Hadza tribesman spent his day walking through the brush, foraging for food. Over the course of a normal day, he consumed between one hundred and one hundred and fifty grams of natural, rough dietary fiber from wild root vegetables, seeds, and berries. He ate twenty or thirty different wild plant types in a single week. His internal garden received a massive, continuous avalanche of prebiotic fertilizer, keeping his helpful workers fed, strong, and multiplying rapidly.

Now, let's be realistic here. I am not telling you that you need to quit your job, sell your house, and move to the East African savanna to hunt wild game with a bow and arrow just to fix your stomach cramps. We live in the modern world, and we enjoy the comforts of indoor plumbing, electricity, and local grocery stores. We are not trying to become historical hunter-gatherers.

What we want to do is take the simple, scientific lesson of the Hadza and adapt it to your neighborhood supermarket aisle. You don't need wild African tubers to feed your gut; you just need to swap out Mark's refined white bagel for a hearty bowl of rolled oats topped with sliced apples and walnuts. You just need to add a can of black beans and some sweet peppers to your Tuesday night taco meat. By deliberately putting rough plant fiber and simple food variety back onto your plate, you can recreate the resilient, resilient gut health of our human ancestors right inside your modern kitchen without ever leaving home.

The Myth Of The Perfect Diet

Before we wrap up our scientific tour of the microbiome and move into your kitchen pantry, we need to address a trap that catches millions of well-meaning people every year. I call it the myth of the perfect diet.

If you scroll through social media or read popular health blogs, you will see self-proclaimed gurus preaching rigid, extreme dieting rules with absolute certainty. One guru swears that a strict Carnivore diet—eating nothing but beef, salt, and water—is the only true way to heal an inflamed gut. Click on the next video, and another expert promises that a strict raw vegan diet—eating nothing but uncooked fruits and vegetables—is the magic cure for every disease on earth. A third expert tells you that you must follow a rigid ketogenic diet, cutting out every single carbohydrate including carrots and apples, if you ever want your digestion to work properly again.

Why do these gurus sound so confident? Because rigid, extreme rules give us a false sense of control when we feel overwhelmed by our health problems. When your stomach is hurting and your energy is tanking, an expert who looks you in the eye and says, "Just stop eating these five foods forever and all your problems will vanish," sounds like a savior.

The problem is that long-term nutritional science paints a very different picture. Rigid, highly restrictive diets might give you a temporary sense of relief for the first few weeks because you are cutting out heavily processed junk food. But over the long haul, extreme exclusion diets actually starve your microbiome and destroy your bacterial diversity.

Think about it logically using everything we just learned about our internal garden. If you go on a strict Carnivore diet and stop eating all plants, what happens to the bacterial families that rely entirely on plant fiber for food? They starve to death and disappear from your garden! When those helpful fiber-eating bugs die off, your gut stops producing those magical anti-inflammatory short-chain fatty acids. Your intestinal wall gets weaker, and your long-term digestive resilience plummets.

The same thing happens if you go on a rigid, fat-free raw diet and exclude all healthy fats and cooked legumes. You starve the bacterial workers who depend on cooked starches and fats, leaving your garden unbalanced and vulnerable.

Here is the liberating truth that the extreme diet gurus don't want you to know. There is no such thing as one single, historically perfect human diet. Human beings have thrived for thousands of years on wildly different diets all across the globe. Traditional populations in the Arctic thrived on diets heavy in fish and sea mammals, while populations in the Mediterranean thrived on diets heavy in olive oil, whole grains, and fresh vegetables. What did all those healthy traditional diets have in common? They were based on whole, unrefined foods eaten in wide variety, without synthetic additives or hyper-processed industrial chemicals.

Stop stressing over whether a carrot has too many carbs, or whether cooking your spinach ruins its enzyme profile. Your gut bacteria do not want you to live in a state of dietary anxiety. In fact, as we learned from the gut-brain axis, stressing out over every single bite of food releases stress hormones that actually impair your digestion and cause bloating!

The best diet for your microbiome is a flexible, relaxed, varied diet made up of real, recognizable grocery store foods that you actually enjoy eating. When you give your body a wide assortment of simple fibers, clean proteins, and healthy fats, your internal master gardeners will gladly handle the rest of the work for you.

Action Step The Plant Count Baseline

Now that you understand the basic rules of your internal garden, it is time to take a baseline reading of where your weekly dietary diversity actually stands right now. Don't worry, this is not a test you can fail, and you are not going to be graded on it. We just need to know your starting point so you can see how much progress you make once we start cooking from the recipe chapters.

We are going to do an exercise called the Plant Count Baseline. Take a piece of paper or open a blank note on your phone. You are going to write down every single plant type you ate over the course of the entire day yesterday—from the moment you woke up to the moment you went to sleep.

Remember our golden rule: a plant is any whole food that grows out of the ground. Be sure to check all six categories! Write down your foods using the simple chart format below:

The Plant Count Baseline Worksheet

Day Evaluated: ______________________________
(Example: Yesterday or Tuesday)

Fruits Eaten

Vegetables Eaten

Whole Grains Eaten

Legumes Eaten

Nuts & Seeds Eaten

Herbs & Spices Eaten

Total Unique Plant Count for the Day

Total Unique Plants: ________

Count each different plant only once, even if you ate it multiple times during the day.

If your total score for yesterday is between three and six different plants, do not feel embarrassed or discouraged. That is exactly where the vast majority of people living in the modern world start out! That low starting number simply explains why your digestive garden has been feeling a little sluggish and overgrown with weeds lately.

Your practical goal as we move through this book is not to jump from five plants a day up to fifty overnight. Your goal is simply to use the upcoming recipes to bump your daily score up by two or three new plants each day until you naturally hit that magical thirty-plants-a-week threshold without even trying. Keep this baseline paper saved in your kitchen so you can look back and celebrate your progress a month from now.

What We Learned About Your Gut Bugs

- **Your gut is a crowded community garden:** You have over thirty-eight trillion microbial workers living inside your lower intestine who digest food, make vitamins, and protect your immune system.
- **Seeds mean nothing without fertilizer:** *Probiotics* are live bacterial seeds, while *prebiotics* are the fibrous plant fertilizers that feed them; swallowing expensive seeds without eating prebiotic plant fertilizer is a complete waste of money.
- **Variety is the golden rule of gut health:** Eating thirty or more different plant types every week—including fruits, vegetables, grains, legumes, nuts, and spices—is the scientifically proven secret to a resilient, healthy microbiome.
- **Your belly talks directly to your brain:** Your gut makes ninety percent of your body's serotonin and communicates constantly with your head via the vagus nerve; healing your intestinal inflammation is a powerful way to relieve anxiety and brain fog.
- **Real food beats rigid dietary dogma:** Extreme diets that cut out entire food groups actually starve your microbiome over time; flexible, varied meals made from simple grocery staples are all your gut workers need to thrive.

The Road Ahead

Take a deep breath and let all that science sink in for a minute. You just learned more about how your body actually works than most people learn in a lifetime, and you did it without needing a medical dictionary or a lab coat. You know who your internal gardeners are, you know what kind of plant fertilizer they love to eat, and you know why ordinary grocery store foods are the ultimate tool for keeping them happy.

Now that we have the biological foundation securely in place, we are done talking about theory. It is time to roll up our sleeves, head into your kitchen, and start putting this science into physical action. In the next chapter, we are going to walk through the ultimate budget-friendly pantry makeover. You are going to learn how to stock your kitchen shelves with cheap, delicious peasant foods that act like high-octane rocket fuel for your microbiome, and how to set up your cooking space so preparing fresh meals feels like a breeze. Grab your shopping list, and let's go transform your kitchen into the happiest gut pharmacy in town.

Chapter 2: The Gut-Healing Pantry Makeover

(On a Budget)

You push your shopping cart down the aisle of a high-end health food store, the kind with soft lighting and employees wearing linen aprons. You pick up a small jar of raw, unpasteurized almond butter. It costs fourteen dollars. You place it in the cart next to a bag of sprouted quinoa and a tiny bottle of cold-pressed green juice.

By the time you reach the register, you have a single brown paper bag of groceries. The cashier smiles and says, "That will be eighty-seven dollars."

Your stomach drops. You swipe your card, walk to your car, and feel a familiar wave of stress. You tell yourself, "Eating healthy is just too expensive. I can't afford to keep this up. It is awful that I have to go broke just to stop my stomach from hurting."

Look, I get it. It is exhausting. But here is the thing. That belief—the idea that healing your digestion requires a massive grocery budget and specialty health stores—is complete nonsense. We do this to ourselves all the time. We build up these rigid rules in our heads. We say we absolutely *must* buy the most expensive, heavily marketed health foods, or we are failing our bodies.

Truth is, the wellness industry wants you to believe that lie. They want you to think that ordinary food is dirty or inadequate.

Wait — actually, no. Let's be completely honest here. The absolute best foods for your microbiome are not found in shiny packages at luxury grocery stores. They are found on the bottom shelves of your local, standard supermarket. They are cheap. They are boring. And they work better than anything else.

The peasant food advantage

Let me introduce you to a concept I call the peasant food advantage.

Historically, the healthiest populations on the planet did not eat artisanal almond butter. They ate what was cheap, what grew easily in the dirt, and what could be stored through the winter. They ate cabbage. They ate oats. They ate dried beans and root vegetables.

These foods are the literal definition of peasant food. And from a biological standpoint, they are absolute superfoods for your gut bacteria.

Let's look at a common green cabbage. A large head of cabbage costs maybe two dollars at a normal grocery store. It is heavy, it lasts for weeks in the fridge, and most people ignore it entirely. But cabbage is packed with a specific type of fiber and compounds called glucosinolates. When these reach your large intestine, your bacteria go crazy for them. They ferment that tough fiber and produce short-chain fatty acids, which directly reduce inflammation in your gut lining.

Now look at dried beans. A one-pound bag of black beans costs about a dollar and fifty cents. That bag contains multiple meals. Beans are loaded with resistant starch. Resistant starch is exactly what it sounds like—it resists human digestion. Your stomach acid cannot break it down. So it travels all the way down to your colon completely intact, acting as the ultimate fertilizer for your good bacteria.

I once worked with a client named David. David was a school teacher, making a modest salary, and he was stressing himself out trying to buy goji berries and hemp seeds to fix his chronic constipation. The financial stress was actually making his digestion worse, because stress shuts down the vagus nerve.

I told him to stop going to the health food store. I sent him to his local supermarket with a ten-dollar bill. I told him to buy a bag of oats, a bag of dried lentils, and a head of cabbage.

At first, he thought I was joking. He felt like he wasn't "doing enough" if he wasn't spending a lot of money. But he followed the plan. He started eating oatmeal for breakfast, lentil stew for lunch, and roasted cabbage with his dinner. Within a week, his digestion regulated. He was spending pennies per meal.

You do not need to be rich to have a healthy stomach. You just need to stop ignoring the cheap stuff.

Navigating the grocery store

You have probably heard the old advice: "Shop the perimeter of the grocery store, because that is where the fresh food is. Avoid the inner aisles."

From what I've seen, this is only half true. Yes, the perimeter has the fresh produce, the meats, and the eggs. You should absolutely spend a good amount of time there.

But if you completely avoid the inner aisles, you are missing out on the cheapest, most effective microbiome fuel available. The inner aisles hold the dried beans, the whole grains, the canned tomatoes, and the spices.

Here is how you actually navigate a normal grocery store without falling into marketing traps.

First, hit the produce section. Do not look for anything exotic. Grab the basics: carrots, onions, garlic, potatoes, broccoli, and apples. These are your heavy hitters.

Next, head into the dry goods aisles. This is where you find the oats, the brown rice, the quinoa, and the dried lentils. The rule here is simple: Look at the ingredient list. If the only ingredient in the bag of oats is "oats," put it in your cart.

Where people get in trouble in the inner aisles is the middle-ground foods. The foods that pretend to be healthy. The boxes of "high-fiber" cereal that contain twenty different unpronounceable chemicals and added sugars. The vegetable chips that are actually just potato starch fried in refined oil.

If it comes in a brightly colored box with a cartoon character or a bold health claim on the front, leave it on the shelf. Real food does not need a marketing team. A bag of black beans doesn't have a slogan.

Your spice rack is medicine

Before you leave the inner aisles, you need to stop at the baking and spice section.

We tend to think of spices just as flavorings. Something you throw in to make a soup taste less boring. But spices are actually densely concentrated plant matter.

Remember the rule from the last section about eating thirty different plants a week? Spices count toward that number.

Spices are incredibly rich in polyphenols. Polyphenols are plant compounds that act like a specialized defense system. When you eat them, the bad bacteria in your gut hate them, but the good bacteria thrive on them.

Oregano, ginger, cinnamon, turmeric, and thyme are powerful gut modulators (Lu et al., 2019). And the best part? A bottle of dried oregano costs three dollars and lasts for months.

When you make a bowl of plain oatmeal, it is just one plant. But if you heavily dash it with cinnamon and nutmeg, you just ate three plants. When you roast chicken, heavily rub it with garlic powder, paprika, and oregano. You are actively feeding your microbiome while making your dinner taste incredible.

The organic perfection myth

This next part? Game-changing. Because I see this specific fear paralyze people every single day.

You are standing in the produce section. You see conventional apples on sale for a dollar a pound. Right next to them are the certified organic apples for three dollars a pound. You read an article once about pesticides and the "Dirty Dozen" list, which claims conventional produce is covered in toxic chemicals.

You look at your budget. You can't afford the organic apples. So, out of fear, you buy no apples at all. You walk away with nothing, telling yourself you are protecting your body.

This drives me nuts.

We build up this rigid, perfectionist belief: "If I cannot eat one hundred percent organic, clean food, then any food I eat is poisoning my gut."

That is awfulizing at its finest. You are taking a minor risk and turning it into a catastrophe. Let's look at the actual science.

Yes, conventional produce uses pesticides. But the residue left on the fruit by the time it reaches your grocery store is incredibly small. The human body, and specifically the liver, is highly adapted to filter out minor environmental toxins.

More importantly, the digestive benefits you get from the fiber and vitamins in a conventional apple far outweigh the microscopic risk of the pesticide residue. Careful risk assessments have found that pesticide residues on conventionally grown produce sit far below levels of concern, and that choosing organic versions of these foods does not meaningfully lower that already negligible risk (Winter & Katz, 2011). Either way, eating plenty of fruits and vegetables, organic or conventional, does far more good for your gut than trace residues could ever do harm.

Eating a conventional carrot is always better than eating no carrot.

If you can afford organic, and you want to buy it, go ahead. But if your budget is tight, do not let perfectionism ruin your progress. Buy the cheap, conventional produce. Take it home. Wash it under running water for twenty seconds. That physical friction removes the vast majority of any remaining residue. Then, eat the food. Stop stressing over it. The stress is worse for your stomach than the conventional apple.

Keep your kitchen simple

You finally get all these cheap groceries home. Now you think you need a massive kitchen setup to process them.

You look online and see wellness influencers using five-hundred-dollar blenders, specialized food processors, and copper cookware. You think, "I can't cook this way, my kitchen is too small and my gear is too cheap."

Again, this won't work for everyone, but between us, you do not need any of that junk.

You need exactly three things to cook gut-healing food.

First, you need one sharp chef's knife. Not a giant block of dull knives. Just one good eight-inch knife. It makes chopping vegetables fast and safe.

Second, you need a large, heavy cutting board. If your cutting board slides around while you chop, put a damp paper towel underneath it.

Third, you need some glass jars or cheap plastic containers to store your leftovers.

That is it. You do not need a fancy blender. You can mash beans with a fork. You can chop cabbage with a knife. You can cook oats in a cheap metal pot you bought at a thrift store. Your gut bacteria do not care how much your cookware costs. They only care about the fiber you send down to them.

Start with a simple swap

We are going to take this one step at a time. I do not want you throwing away everything in your pantry today. That is a great way to waste money and get overwhelmed.

Instead, the next time you go to the grocery store, we are going to make five simple, cheap swaps. We are going to replace refined, low-fiber foods with their peasant-food equivalents. This doesn't require a lot of money or a lot of effort. It just requires making a different choice in the same aisle.

Action Step: The 5-Item Pantry Swap

The next time you go grocery shopping, make these five simple swaps to support a healthier gut. Small changes like these can significantly increase your fiber intake without completely changing the way you eat.

1. Swap White Rice for Brown Rice or Quinoa

Brown rice and quinoa contain significantly more fiber than white rice, helping to nourish your gut microbes while keeping you fuller for longer.

2. Swap Instant Sugary Oatmeal for Plain Rolled Oats

Choose plain rolled oats instead of flavored instant packets. Add your own cinnamon, fruit, nuts, or seeds at home for natural sweetness and extra nutrients.

3. Swap Regular Wheat Pasta for Red Lentil or Chickpea Pasta

These legume-based pastas cook much like traditional pasta but provide substantially more protein and fiber, making them a simple upgrade for everyday meals.

4. Swap Canned Soup for Canned Black Beans

Keep canned black beans in your pantry for a quick, affordable meal. Simply rinse, heat, and season with your favorite spices—such as taco seasoning—for an easy, fiber-rich option.

5. Swap Potato Chips for Air-Popped Popcorn

Air-popped popcorn is a whole grain that's naturally high in fiber. Season it with herbs or spices instead of butter-heavy toppings for a satisfying, gut-friendly snack.

Key takeaways

- The most powerful gut-healing foods are cheap, accessible staples like cabbage, beans, oats, and potatoes.
- Avoid the middle-ground processed foods with health claims; stick to the produce section and the single-ingredient dry goods aisles.
- Spices are concentrated plant matter packed with polyphenols; use them heavily to increase your daily plant count.
- Do not let the fear of conventional produce stop you from eating vegetables. Washing conventional produce is perfectly safe and biologically superior to avoiding vegetables altogether.
- You do not need expensive kitchen gadgets to cook well; a single sharp knife and a cutting board are enough to change your diet.

Speaking of which, once you get these cheap, high-fiber foods home, there is a very specific way you need to eat them. Because if you just open a can of beans, dump them on a massive pile of cabbage, and eat it all at once, you are going to be in for a terrible night. Let's talk about why healthy food sometimes hurts, and how to stop the bloating before it starts.

Chapter 3: The "Low and Slow" Fiber Protocol

You made the swaps. You stopped buying the expensive powders. You went to the store and bought broccoli, black beans, lentils, and rolled oats. You are feeling incredibly motivated.

You get home, chop up a massive salad of raw kale, dump half a can of chickpeas on top, add some raw onions, and eat the whole bowl. You feel proud of yourself.

Two hours later, you are lying on your couch in the fetal position. Your stomach is distended. You look six months pregnant. The gas pain is sharp, trapping itself under your ribs.

You think, "Well, that proves it. My body is broken. I can't handle fiber. Every time I eat healthy food, I feel awful. I might as well just go back to eating white toast and taking pills."

This is the exact moment where ninety percent of people quit.

I get it. It is intensely frustrating to do exactly what the experts tell you to do, only to end up in physical pain. We tell ourselves that healthy food should immediately make us feel healthy. When it doesn't, we assume we have a permanent medical condition.

But here is the reality. Your body isn't broken. Your gut bacteria are just wildly out of shape.

When healthy food hurts

Think about your microbiome like a muscle.

Imagine a guy who hasn't been to the gym in ten years. He spends his days sitting at a desk. One day, he decides to get healthy. He walks into a gym, loads three hundred pounds onto a barbell, and tries to squat it.

What happens? He collapses. His muscles tear. He is in agony for a week.

Did he fail because squats are inherently bad for humans? No. He failed because he asked a weak, untrained muscle to handle a massive load with zero preparation.

Your gut works the exact same way. If you have been eating a standard Western diet—low in fiber, high in processed foods—for years, the specific bacteria required to break down heavy fiber have died off or gone dormant.

When you suddenly drop forty grams of raw fiber into your digestive tract, you do not have the microbial workforce to handle it.

Why fermentation feels like a balloon

To understand why this hurts so much, we need to look at how digestion actually happens.

When you eat a piece of chicken, your human stomach acid and enzymes break it down relatively quickly. It is mostly absorbed in the small intestine.

But when you eat a chickpea, the fiber survives the stomach acid. It moves all the way down to your large intestine. There, your bacteria eat it. The way they eat it is through a process called *fermentation.*

When bacteria ferment fiber, they release two things. First, they release those incredibly healing short-chain fatty acids we talked about earlier. Second, they release gas.

Gas is a completely normal, healthy byproduct of fermentation. A healthy person passes gas around ten times a day on average, and up to roughly twenty times still sits comfortably within the normal range (Furne & Levitt, 1996).

But if you drop a massive amount of fiber into an untrained gut, the few bacteria you *do* have go into overdrive. They ferment the food rapidly, producing a huge spike in gas. Because your gut motility—the muscle contractions that move things along—is likely sluggish from years of poor diet, that gas gets trapped.

It acts exactly like a balloon inflating inside your abdomen. That is why your pants suddenly don't fit by 4:00 PM.

The raw kale disaster

Let me tell you about Jessica. Jessica was thirty-four, constantly exhausted, and dealing with daily bloating. She read that raw vegan diets heal the gut, so she went all in.

On day one, she ate a massive raw kale salad with broccoli florets and raw pumpkin seeds. By the afternoon, she called me in tears. She said, "I am doing everything right, but I feel like my stomach is tearing apart."

I told her to stop immediately. We completely changed her approach. I told her no raw vegetables for the next two weeks.

Instead of a raw kale salad, I had her eat half a cup of thoroughly cooked spinach. Instead of raw broccoli, I had her eat roasted carrots.

Why? Because cooking is a form of pre-digestion. When you boil or roast a vegetable, the heat breaks down the tough cellular walls of the plant. It softens the fiber. By the time it reaches your bacteria, it is much easier for them to ferment. It produces a slow, steady release of gas rather than an explosive one.

Jessica pivoted to cooked vegetables. The pain stopped immediately. A month later, as her bacterial workforce grew stronger, she was able to handle raw salads again without any bloating.

The four week fiber protocol

You cannot rush this process. We have to train your gut muscle slowly.

Most health guidelines suggest adults need roughly thirty grams of dietary fiber a day. The average person currently eats about fifteen grams. If you try to double your intake overnight, you will suffer.

Instead, we are going to use the "Low and Slow" protocol. We are going to scale up your fiber so gently that your body barely notices the change, giving your bacteria time to multiply and adapt.

Week 1: The cooked baseline For the first seven days, do not change how much you eat. Just change *how* you prepare it. Avoid all raw vegetables. No big salads. Cook all your vegetables until they are fork-tender. Roast your carrots, steam your zucchini, sauté your spinach. If you eat fruit, stick to softer fruits like berries or bananas, rather than tough raw apples with the skin on.

Week 2: The three gram bump Now, we add just three to five extra grams of fiber to your daily total. That is a very small amount. It is equal to adding half an apple, or two tablespoons of chia seeds, to your breakfast. Continue to cook most of your vegetables. You can introduce very small amounts of soft beans, like red lentils, which are much easier to digest than kidney beans.

Week 3: The crunch returns Add another three to five grams. Now you can start introducing raw, crunchy vegetables back into your routine. Have a small side salad with your dinner. Leave the skin on your baked potato. Your bacteria have spent two weeks multiplying; they are now strong enough to handle raw cellular walls.

Week 4: Reaching the goal Add a final three to five grams. By now, you should be comfortably eating close to thirty grams of fiber a day. You can introduce heavier beans, like black beans and chickpeas. You will notice that your bowel movements are regular and the painful, trapped gas is gone.

Water is non negotiable

There is a major catch to this entire process. You can follow the four-week protocol perfectly, but if you fail on this next step, it will not work.

Fiber acts like a sponge in your digestive tract.

Imagine taking a dry kitchen sponge and trying to push it through a plastic tube. It will get stuck. It will drag. It will cause a massive blockage.

Now imagine soaking that same sponge in water. It becomes soft, pliable, and slides right through the tube.

When you increase your fiber intake, you absolutely must increase your water intake. If you eat a massive bowl of oats and beans but only drink one glass of water all day, that fiber turns into concrete in your intestines. It will cause severe constipation.

You need to drink enough water so that your urine is pale yellow. Do not obsess over drinking exactly a gallon a day. Just drink a large glass of water with every meal, and sip throughout the day.

Chew your food

Quick side note, because we all do this.

You come home from work. You are starving. You heat up a plate of food, stand over the sink or sit in front of the television, and you inhale the meal in five minutes.

We swallow our food almost entirely whole.

Digestion does not start in your stomach. It starts in your mouth. Your saliva contains an enzyme called *amylase*, which specifically breaks down carbohydrates and starches. Furthermore, the physical act of chewing crushes the food, exposing more surface area for your stomach acid to work on.

If you swallow a piece of broccoli whole, your stomach acid has to work incredibly hard to break it down. By the time it reaches your large intestine, it is still in large, unmanageable chunks. Your bacteria struggle to ferment it, which leads to—you guessed it—more gas.

Look, we all eat over the sink sometimes. But you have to slow down. Try putting your fork down between bites. Chew your food until it is the consistency of applesauce before you swallow. It feels unnatural at first, but it is one of the fastest ways to eliminate post-meal bloating.

How to cook a bean

Before I forget, we need to talk about beans. Beans are the cheapest, most effective gut food on the planet, but they are also the most notorious for causing gas.

There is a biological reason for this. Beans contain a specific type of carbohydrate called *oligosaccharides*. Humans do not have the enzyme to break this down. It goes straight to your bacteria, and they ferment it rapidly.

But you can drastically reduce the oligosaccharides before the bean ever enters your mouth.

If you buy canned beans, do not just open the can and dump the contents into a pan. That thick, cloudy liquid in the can is concentrated oligosaccharides. Pour the beans into a strainer and rinse them under cold running water until the water runs completely clear and all the foam is gone. That one step removes a massive amount of the gas-causing compounds.

If you are cooking dried beans, you must soak them. The best method is the hot soak. Put your dried beans in a large pot, cover them with water, and boil them for three minutes. Then, turn off the heat, cover the pot, and let them sit for four hours.

After four hours, pour the water down the drain. Do not cook the beans in their soaking water. Rinse them thoroughly, add fresh water to the pot, and cook them until they are completely soft. If a bean is slightly crunchy, it will destroy your stomach. They must be creamy all the way through.

This isn't just a cooking tip. It is a digestive requirement.

We have covered a lot of ground here. You know how to shop, and you know how to eat the food without inflating like a balloon. It is time to see exactly where you stand today.

Action Step: Establish Your Fiber Baseline

Before making any changes to your fiber intake, it's helpful to understand where you're starting.

Step 1: Review Your Plant Tally

Look back at the Plant Tally you completed in Chapter 1, based on everything you ate yesterday.

Step 2: Estimate Your Fiber Intake

Roughly calculate your total fiber intake for the day. You don't need to be exact—an estimate is enough.

Quick reference:

- 1 slice of white bread ≈ **1 g** of fiber
- 1 medium apple ≈ **4 g** of fiber
- 1 cup of beans ≈ **15 g** of fiber

Step 3: Record Your Baseline

Write down your estimated total fiber intake for the day:

My estimated daily fiber intake: _______ g

Step 4: Follow Your Week 1 Goal

If your estimated fiber intake is **under 15 g per day, do not increase it yet**. Your goal for **Week 1** is to keep your fiber intake at approximately the same level while ensuring that **all vegetables are thoroughly cooked**.

Step 5: Prepare for Week 2

Next week, you'll increase your daily fiber intake by **just 3 grams**. This is a small, gradual increase—for example, adding **half an apple** or another food that provides approximately **3 g of fiber**.

This version is structured for easy reading while keeping the instructions clear and actionable.

Final thoughts

- Bloating after eating healthy food does not mean your body is broken; it means your gut bacteria are untrained and overwhelmed.
- Cooking vegetables softens their tough cellular walls, acting as a form of pre-digestion that dramatically reduces gas and bloating.
- You must scale your fiber intake up slowly, using a four-week protocol, to allow your microbiome time to multiply and adapt.
- Increasing dietary fiber without simultaneously increasing water intake will lead to severe constipation.
- Properly chewing your food and thoroughly rinsing canned beans are simple, mechanical habits that drastically reduce the amount of gas produced during digestion.

Chapter 4: Stealth Fermentation

(Probiotics for Haters)

You stand in front of your open refrigerator, staring at a fourteen-dollar jar of artisanal kimchi. You unscrew the lid. The smell hits you immediately — a sharp, sour, sulfurous punch to the nose. You physically recoil. You try to take a bite, but the texture of the fermented cabbage makes you gag. You spit it out, screw the lid back on, and shove the jar to the dark back corner of the fridge, right next to last year's mustard.

You close the fridge and let out a long sigh. You think, "I just can't do it. I hate fermented food. My gut is never going to heal because I can't force myself to eat this awful stuff."

I get it. It is exhausting trying to choke down food that your taste buds actively reject.

But here is the thing. You are falling into a classic mental trap. You are telling yourself that because you hate the taste of sauerkraut and kimchi, your situation is entirely hopeless. You think you *must* eat foods you despise in order to be healthy. That is simply irrational.

Truth is, nobody is forcing you to eat straight from a jar of sour cabbage. You do not have to develop a taste for strong fermented foods to rebuild your microbiome. We just have to get a little bit sneaky.

Surviving the acid wash

Before we talk about hiding these foods, we need to understand why we are even bothering. If you hate fermented foods, why not just go back to taking the expensive probiotic pill we talked about in the introduction?

It comes down to survival. Your stomach is a hostile environment. It is filled with hydrochloric acid designed to break down food and kill invading pathogens. When you swallow an isolated probiotic capsule with a glass of water on an empty stomach, that gelatin capsule dissolves very quickly. The billions of naked bacteria are suddenly dumped into a pool of burning acid.

A massive percentage of them die instantly. They never even make it to your large intestine, which is where they actually do their work.

But food-based probiotics are different. When you eat a fermented food, those good bacteria are wrapped in a protective *food matrix*. They are buffered by proteins, fats, and fibers.

When bacteria are consumed within a dairy or plant-based matrix, their survival rate through gastric juices is significantly higher than when consumed in isolated powder forms (Marco et al., 2017).

Eating your probiotics ensures they actually survive the trip. You get more living bacteria to your lower intestine from a single spoonful of fermented food than you do from a fifty-dollar bottle of pills.

The stealth approach

So, how do we get that spoonful into your body if you hate the taste of sour food? We use the stealth approach.

We stop treating fermented foods as the star of the meal. We stop putting giant, intimidating piles of sauerkraut next to our eggs. Instead, we use fermented foods as background ingredients. We blend them, mask them, and hide them inside flavors you already love.

You probably eat foods all the time without realizing exactly what is in them. If you love restaurant salad dressings, you are usually eating a base of mayonnaise or buttermilk. If you enjoy a thick, creamy smoothie, you are often drinking a hidden banana that provides the texture.

We are going to do the exact same thing with probiotics. We are going to hijack your daily meals and turn them into probiotic delivery systems without altering the taste you expect.

Kefir versus yogurt

Let's start with the easiest swap in the grocery store. Most people know that yogurt contains probiotics. But yogurt is actually a lightweight when it comes to gut health.

Standard grocery store yogurt might contain two or three strains of good bacteria. That is fine, but it is not going to radically change your internal garden.

Kefir is different. Kefir is a fermented milk drink. It looks like thin yogurt, but it is a biological powerhouse. While yogurt has two or three strains of bacteria, kefir contains up to sixty different strains of bacteria and beneficial yeasts. It is one of the most potent probiotic foods on earth.

But there is a catch. Plain kefir tastes extremely tart. If you drink a glass of it straight, it tastes like sour milk.

So, we don't drink it straight.

Instead, you use plain, unsweetened kefir as the liquid base for your morning smoothie. When you blend half a cup of kefir with a handful of sweet frozen blueberries, half a banana, and a spoonful of peanut butter, the sour taste completely vanishes. The sweetness of the fruit entirely masks the tartness of the dairy. You are drinking billions of live, diverse bacteria, and it tastes exactly like a normal berry milkshake.

You can also use kefir in place of buttermilk to make homemade ranch dressing. When mixed with garlic powder, onion powder, and fresh dill, the tartness of the kefir just tastes like the expected tang of a good ranch. You pour it over your salad, and suddenly your lunch is actively healing your gut.

Miso as a secret weapon

Now, let's talk about savory foods.

I once worked with a guy named Tom. Tom was a construction manager in his fifties. He was a meat-and-potatoes guy. He suffered from terrible acid reflux and bloating, but if I even mentioned the word "fermented," he would roll his eyes. He absolutely refused to eat yogurt, kefir, or cabbage.

I told him I had a secret ingredient that would make his favorite foods taste better, and he just had to promise to use it. I introduced him to white miso paste.

Miso is a traditional Japanese paste made from fermented soybeans. Most people only know it from the cloudy soup they get at sushi restaurants. But miso is not just for soup. It is one of the most versatile ingredients in your kitchen.

White miso is fermented for a short time, making it mild and slightly sweet. But more importantly, it is packed with *umami*. Umami is the deep, savory, salty flavor that makes things like roasted meat, parmesan cheese, and mushrooms taste so good.

Tom loved making mashed potatoes. I told him to boil his potatoes and mash them with butter as usual, but instead of adding a heavy pinch of salt at the end, I told him to stir in a tablespoon of white miso paste.

He was incredibly skeptical. He thought I was trying to ruin his potatoes. But he tried it. The miso melted into the warm potatoes. It didn't taste like sushi soup. It just tasted like the richest, most savory, deeply comforting mashed potatoes he had ever eaten.

He started putting a spoonful of white miso into his pan gravies. He whisked it into his olive oil to dress his roasted vegetables. He was eating massive amounts of live probiotics every single day, and he was doing it while eating his favorite comfort foods.

The heat warning

This brings us to a critical rule. If you mess this up, you ruin the entire stealth approach.

Heat kills bacteria.

If you take a scoop of live miso paste and throw it into a pot of boiling water on the stove, you will instantly kill every single beneficial microbe in the paste. It will still taste good, but it will be biologically dead. You will get zero probiotic benefit.

The same goes for kefir, sauerkraut, or any other live food.

You must always add your fermented foods at the very end of the cooking process, off the direct heat.

If you are making a stew and want to add miso, you cook the stew completely. You turn off the stove. You ladle a little bit of the warm (not boiling) broth into a small bowl, whisk the miso into that bowl until it dissolves, and then stir it back into the warm pot.

If you are putting a spoonful of sauerkraut into a bowl of warm chili, you add it to the bowl sitting on your table, not the pot boiling on the stove.

We want the food to be warm enough to be comforting, but not so hot that it acts as an antibiotic.

This won't work perfectly the first time you try it. You might add too much miso and make something too salty. You might use too much kefir and make a smoothie too tart. That is okay. You won't master this overnight.

But you have to stop telling yourself that you are incapable of eating probiotics just because you dislike the strong, raw flavors. You are in control of your kitchen. You get to decide how these foods taste.

Action Step: The Miso Swap

Add more flavor—and beneficial fermented foods—to your meals with this simple swap.

1. Buy a small tub of **white miso paste** from the grocery store. It's usually found in the refrigerated section near the tofu or other refrigerated plant-based products.
2. The next time you prepare a savory meal—such as roasted vegetables, rice, soup, or mashed potatoes—leave the salt shaker aside.
3. Once the food is fully cooked and removed from the heat, stir in **1 teaspoon of white miso paste**.
4. Mix until the miso is fully dissolved and evenly distributed.
5. Taste your meal and notice the rich, savory umami flavor that miso adds while reducing the need for extra salt.

Takeaways for Chapter 4

- Food-based probiotics survive stomach acid much better than supplement pills because the food matrix physically protects the bacteria.
- You do not have to eat raw, sour foods to get probiotic benefits; you can seamlessly hide fermented ingredients inside familiar meals.
- Kefir contains significantly more bacterial strains than standard yogurt and can easily be hidden in fruit smoothies or savory salad dressings.
- White miso paste acts as a powerful, savory salt replacement that adds umami flavor and live bacteria to everyday comfort foods.
- Never subject live fermented foods to boiling heat, as this instantly kills the beneficial bacteria; always stir them into warm dishes off the stove.

Before I forget, hiding probiotics is a great strategy for lunch and dinner, but we need to talk about the most chaotic part of your day. The time when you are rushing out the door and your dietary choices are usually driven by pure panic. Let's head into your morning routine.

Chapter 5: Breakfasts That Wake Up Your Microbiome

(Recipes)

It is 7:15 AM on a Tuesday. You hit snooze twice. You are running late. You rush into the kitchen, pour a cup of black coffee, and grab whatever is fast. Maybe it is a heavily processed granola bar wrapped in plastic. Maybe it is a bowl of sugary cereal. Or maybe you skip food entirely, living on caffeine and adrenaline until lunchtime.

You tell yourself, "I just don't have time to cook a healthy breakfast in the morning."

This drives me nuts too. We all feel the time crunch. But skipping breakfast or relying on processed sugar to wake up is setting a disastrous tone for your digestion for the rest of the day.

When you wake up, your gut bacteria wake up. They have been fasting all night. They are hungry, and they are waiting for instructions.

If the first thing you send down to them is refined sugar and caffeine, you trigger a massive spike in your blood sugar. That spike leads to an inevitable crash a few hours later. More importantly, refined sugars actually feed the bad, inflammatory bacteria in your gut while leaving your good bacteria completely starved.

Look, telling yourself you don't have time is just an excuse to avoid changing a bad habit. You do have time. You just need a better system. We are going to build breakfasts that wake up your microbiome, keep your blood sugar stable, and require almost zero effort on a busy Tuesday morning.

Breaking the fast with fiber

The primary goal of your first meal is incredibly simple: You must break your fast with fiber.

When you eat a breakfast rich in complex fiber—like oats, seeds, or heavy whole grains—you create a physical mesh in your stomach. This mesh slows down the rate at which your body absorbs sugars. It keeps your energy stable, prevents the mid-morning crash, and immediately delivers fertilizer to your large intestine.

Consuming a high-fiber breakfast significantly alters the gut microbiome's daily rhythms, leading to improved glycemic control and sustained energy throughout the day (Zeevi et al., 2015).

If you start the day with fiber, you put a protective shield over your digestion. You are significantly less likely to experience painful bloating after lunch and dinner because you have already primed the engine.

The sweet versus savory debate

When we think of breakfast in the Western world, we usually think of sweet foods. Pancakes, waffles, muffins, sweetened yogurts.

From a biological standpoint, this is a terrible idea. Starting the day with sweet foods, even natural sweets like honey or large amounts of fruit, can still spike your blood sugar if there is not enough protein and fiber to anchor it down.

Savory breakfasts are often superior for gut health. A savory breakfast might look like a bowl of leftover lentils, a spinach scramble, or a slice of dense sourdough bread topped with avocado and pumpkin seeds. Savory meals naturally lean toward vegetables and healthy fats, which keep your digestion smooth.

That said, I know some people simply cannot stomach the idea of eating beans or spinach at 7:00 AM. If you demand a sweet breakfast, you can absolutely have it. But you must construct it properly. You have to anchor the sweetness with massive amounts of prebiotic fiber.

Morning recipes that actually work

In the complete cookbook, there are 15 dedicated breakfast recipes. We include options for every palate. There are *Savory Miso Spinach Scrambles*, *Prebiotic Berry Smash Toasts*, *Hidden-Veggie Frittatas*, and *Gut-Healing Grain Bowls*.

But right now, I want to give you the blueprints for the three most effective, time-saving breakfasts you can possibly make. These are the heavy hitters.

1. The Kefir Overnight Oats (Sweet & Fast) This is the ultimate anchor breakfast. You make it the night before, meaning it takes exactly zero minutes to prepare in the morning.

- **The Base:** Half a cup of plain, rolled oats. (Prebiotic fiber).
- **The Liquid:** Half a cup of plain kefir. (Massive live probiotics).
- **The Crunch:** One tablespoon of chia seeds and one tablespoon of chopped walnuts. (Polyphenols and healthy fats).
- **The Sweetness:** A handful of frozen blueberries and a heavy dash of cinnamon.
- **How it works:** You put all of this in a glass jar, stir it up, and leave it in the fridge overnight. The oats soften in the kefir. The chia seeds expand, creating a pudding-like texture. In the morning, you just grab a spoon and eat it. You get massive fiber, zero refined sugar, and stealthy probiotics.

2. The 5-Minute Bean and Egg Skillet (Savory & Warm) If you need a hot meal, you do not have time to bake an intricate casserole. You need speed.

- **The Base:** Half a cup of canned black beans (rinsed well) and half a cup of cherry tomatoes.
- **The Protein:** Two whole eggs.
- **The Flavor:** A pinch of cumin, oregano, and salt.
- **How it works:** Put a small pan on the stove with a splash of olive oil. Toss in the beans and tomatoes until they are warm and the tomatoes start to blister. Crack the two eggs directly over the beans. Cover the pan with a lid for three minutes until the eggs are cooked. Slide it onto a plate. You just ate massive amounts of resistant starch and protein in five minutes flat.

3. The Prebiotic Berry Smash Toast (Crunchy & Satisfying)
Sometimes you just want toast. But white bread and jam is a blood sugar disaster.

- **The Base:** One thick slice of real sourdough bread. (Sourdough undergoes a fermentation process that pre-digests the gluten, making it much easier on your stomach).
- **The Spread:** Two tablespoons of plain almond butter or mashed avocado.
- **The Smash:** Take a handful of fresh raspberries, put them in a small bowl, and literally smash them with a fork until they look like jam.
- **The Topping:** Spread the nut butter on the toasted sourdough, top it with the smashed raspberries, and sprinkle heavily with hemp seeds.
- **How it works:** You get the psychological comfort of toast and jam, but you are actually eating complex fermented carbohydrates, healthy fats, and raw fruit fiber.

Batch cooking for reality

Let me tell you about Maria. Maria had three kids under the age of ten. Her mornings were absolute chaos. She told me, "I love the idea of cooking eggs and beans, but I barely have time to tie my own shoes before I have to get the kids in the car."

She felt totally defeated. She was living on cold leftover toast from her kids' plates.

I told her to stop trying to cook on weekday mornings. It was an irrational demand she was placing on herself.

Instead, we implemented Sunday batch cooking. On Sunday afternoon, when the house was slightly calmer, Maria took five empty glass jars. She lined them up on the counter. She filled all five jars with the Kefir Overnight Oats recipe. It took her exactly ten minutes to measure the oats, pour the kefir, drop in the frozen berries, and screw the lids on.

She put all five jars in the fridge.

On Monday morning, she didn't have to think. She didn't have to cook. She just opened the fridge, grabbed a jar, and ate it while she was packing her kids' backpacks. She got 30 grams of diverse plants and massive probiotics before 8:00 AM, with zero stress.

You won't master your mornings perfectly every day. Sometimes you will oversleep. Sometimes you will end up eating a bagel at the office. That is fine. But if you have a system in place, you remove the daily friction of trying to make good choices while half-asleep.

Action Step: The Sunday Prep

Set yourself up for an easier week by preparing breakfast in advance.

1. Choose one no-cook breakfast recipe, such as **Kefir Overnight Oats**, that can be made ahead of time.
2. Buy the ingredients during your regular grocery shopping trip.
3. On Sunday evening, gather three jars or food containers.
4. Prepare three servings of your chosen breakfast at the same time and store them in the refrigerator.

5. For the first three days of your work week, simply grab a prepared breakfast and enjoy. Pay attention to how much time and mental energy you save by having one less decision to make each morning.

Takeaways for Chapter 5

- Breaking your overnight fast with fiber stabilizes your blood sugar and provides immediate fuel for your resting gut bacteria.
- Relying on refined sugars and processed bars in the morning feeds inflammatory bacteria and guarantees a severe energy crash later in the day.
- Savory breakfasts naturally lean toward gut-healing vegetables and healthy fats, but sweet breakfasts are effective if anchored by dense fibers like oats and chia seeds.
- Properly made sourdough bread is easier to digest than standard white bread because the fermentation process pre-digests heavy starches.
- Batch-cooking cold breakfasts on the weekend removes the stress of weekday mornings, making consistency nearly effortless.

Quick side note, nailing breakfast is a massive win, but it only sets the stage. By the time 2:00 PM rolls around, you are going to face a completely different biological challenge. Let's talk about the meal that usually destroys your afternoon productivity, and how to fix it.

Chapter 6: Lunches for Midday Energy

(Recipes)

It is 2:30 PM. You are sitting at your desk, staring blankly at your computer monitor. You read the same email three times, but the words aren't making any sense. Your eyelids feel like they weigh ten pounds each. A heavy, sluggish fog has settled over your brain.

You think back to what you ate for lunch. You tried to be so good. You went to the deli across the street and ordered a garden salad. Just iceberg lettuce, a few slices of pale cucumber, some grilled chicken, and a fat-free vinaigrette.

You tell yourself, "I ate a healthy salad! I should feel vibrant and energetic. Why do I feel like I need a three-hour nap under my desk?"

Here is what I noticed. We have been brainwashed into believing that the ultimate healthy lunch is a plate of plain, raw leaves. We call this the "sad desk salad."

Truth is, the sad desk salad is an absolute disaster for your midday energy.

Escaping the sad desk salad trap

Let's look at the biology of that salad. Iceberg lettuce is essentially crunchy water. It contains almost zero calories, very little complex fiber, and barely any nutrients. The grilled chicken provides protein, which is fine, but your brain does not run on protein. Your brain runs on glucose derived from complex carbohydrates.

When you eat a sad desk salad, you are severely under-fueling your body. You give your brain no usable energy.

Simultaneously, you give your microbiome nothing to ferment. Without dense, complex fibers to chew on, your gut bacteria sit idle.

Because the gut and the brain are connected by the vagus nerve, an under-fueled, idle gut sends lethargy signals straight to your brain.

That 2:00 PM brain fog is not a lack of caffeine. It is a lack of complex carbohydrates and prebiotic fiber.

If you want to survive the afternoon without crashing, you have to stop eating meals that look like rabbit food. You need meals with structural integrity. You need meals that take your body hours to break down, providing a slow, steady drip of energy into your bloodstream.

The anatomy of a gut-healthy bowl

We are going to abandon the traditional salad. Instead, we are going to build gut-healthy bowls.

In the complete cookbook, we provide 15 specific midday recipes to keep you moving. There are *Hidden-Kraut Turkey Wraps*, *10-Minute Chickpea Mash Sandwiches*, and *Leftover-Makeover Grain Bowls*.

But you do not always need a strict recipe. You just need a framework. A properly constructed gut-healthy bowl follows a very specific anatomy. Once you memorize this five-part structure, you can build a perfect lunch out of whatever happens to be sitting in your fridge.

- **1. The Base (Complex Carbohydrate):** This is your energy anchor. Instead of lettuce, start with half a cup of cooked quinoa, brown rice, farro, or roasted sweet potatoes. This provides the slow-burning glucose your brain desperately needs at 2:00 PM.
- **2. The Veg (Fiber and Color):** Add a massive handful of vegetables. But aim for density. Roasted carrots, steamed broccoli, chopped bell peppers, or shredded purple cabbage.

- **3. The Protein (Satiety):** This keeps you full. Leftover roasted chicken, a hard-boiled egg, half a cup of rinsed black beans, or baked tofu.
- **4. The Ferment (The Probiotic Hit):** This is where you heal the gut. A spoonful of sauerkraut, a scoop of kimchi, or a drizzle of miso dressing.
- **5. The Crunch (Polyphenols and Fats):** Texture matters for psychological satisfaction. A sprinkle of pumpkin seeds, chopped walnuts, or slivered almonds.

When you put these five elements together, you create a meal that is physically heavy. It is dense. It takes your human stomach a long time to break down the protein and the base. By the time the meal reaches your large intestine, your bacteria have a massive feast of diverse fibers and polyphenols to ferment.

You feel full, but you do not feel sluggish.

Meals rich in complex, slow-fermenting dietary fibers maintain postprandial blood glucose stability and prevent the acute cognitive fatigue often associated with low-fiber, low-carbohydrate midday meals (Slavin, 2013).

Midday recipes to keep you moving

Let's look at how this framework translates into real, fast recipes.

Take the **10-Minute Chickpea Mash Sandwich**. I love this one because it completely replaces the need for highly processed deli meats, which are terrible for gut inflammation. You take a can of chickpeas, rinse them well to remove the gas-causing sugars, and throw them in a bowl. You take a fork and mash them up until they look like tuna salad. You stir in a spoonful of plain kefir or Greek yogurt, a squeeze of lemon juice, some chopped celery, and a heavy pinch of dill. Scoop that mash onto two slices of dense sourdough bread. You just made a lunch packed with resistant starch, plant protein, and stealth probiotics, all in under ten minutes.

Or consider the **Leftover-Makeover Grain Bowl**. The night before, you made chicken and roasted broccoli for dinner. You deliberately cooked a little extra. The next morning, you put a scoop of cooked quinoa in a glass container. You add the leftover chicken and broccoli. Then—and this is the secret—you add a massive spoonful of raw sauerkraut to the corner of the container. You pack it for lunch. It took two minutes to assemble, but it hits all five points of the anatomy framework.

Dressings as a delivery system

This brings me to my favorite trick in the entire book.

If you are packing lunches for work, you need flavor. Most people reach for bottled dressings from the grocery store. I want you to go to your fridge right now and look at the back of your favorite bottled salad dressing.

The first ingredient is almost certainly a refined seed oil, like soybean or canola oil. The second ingredient is usually sugar or high fructose corn syrup. Then you will find a long list of emulsifiers and preservatives.

These bottled dressings are like pouring gasoline on a fire if you have an inflamed gut. Emulsifiers, specifically, have been shown to directly damage the mucosal lining of the intestines.

We are going to replace that garbage with a dressing that actively heals you. We are going to make **Probiotic Ranch**.

I mentioned this briefly in the previous chapter, but here is the exact science of why it works. You take half a cup of plain kefir (your probiotic powerhouse). You mix it with a tablespoon of olive oil (healthy fats). You add garlic powder, onion powder, dried dill, and a pinch of salt (polyphenols and flavor).

You shake it up in a small jar. It takes sixty seconds to make.

When you pour this over your lunch bowl, you are not just adding flavor. You are delivering a liquid wave of living bacteria straight into your digestive tract, perfectly paired with the complex fiber in your bowl. The bacteria eat the fiber, multiply, and heal the gut lining.

Safe storage and heating

Now, there is a very practical hurdle here.

I had a client named David who was doing great with his meal preps. He built perfect gut-healthy bowls with roasted sweet potatoes, chicken, and a big scoop of kimchi. He took his glass container to the office.

At noon, he put the entire container in the office microwave and hit the three-minute button. He sat down and ate a steaming hot bowl of food.

He was incredibly frustrated when he didn't see any improvement in his digestion.

I asked him to walk me through exactly what he did. When he told me about the microwave, I stopped him.

Wait — actually, no. We just talked about this in Chapter 4. Heat kills bacteria.

When David microwaved his entire bowl, he superheated the kimchi. He instantly vaporized billions of beneficial probiotic strains. He turned a gut-healing superfood into dead cabbage.

If you pack a lunch that contains a live fermented food—like kimchi, sauerkraut, or a kefir dressing—you cannot microwave it.

You have two options.

Option one: Eat the bowl cold. Grains, roasted vegetables, and proteins taste fantastic cold or at room temperature if they are properly seasoned.

Option two: Separate the hot from the cold. If you must have a warm lunch, put your quinoa and chicken in a microwave-safe container. Put your sauerkraut and probiotic dressing in a tiny separate plastic cup. Microwave the main container. When it is hot, take it out, and then stir in the cold kraut and dressing.

It takes an extra five seconds of planning, but it ensures your internal garden actually receives the seeds you are trying to plant.

This won't work perfectly every time. You might forget and microwave the dressing once or twice. That is fine. Don't awfulize it. Just try to remember for the next day.

Action Step: Make Probiotic Ranch Dressing

This quick homemade dressing is an easy way to add probiotics to your lunch every day.

You'll Need

- ½ cup plain, unsweetened kefir
- 1 tablespoon olive oil
- ½ teaspoon garlic powder
- ½ teaspoon onion powder
- ½ teaspoon dried dill
- A pinch of salt
- A pinch of black pepper

Instructions

1. Pour the kefir and olive oil into a small glass jar with a tight-fitting lid.
2. Add the garlic powder, onion powder, dried dill, salt, and black pepper.

3. Secure the lid and shake vigorously for about 10 seconds, until well combined.
4. Store the dressing in the refrigerator.

Daily Habit

Keep the jar in your work refrigerator (or at home if you work remotely) and pour it over salads, grain bowls, roasted vegetables, or wraps to add a convenient serving of probiotics to your lunch.

Takeaways for Chapter 6

- The "sad desk salad" consisting of plain lettuce and lean protein lacks the complex carbohydrates required to fuel your brain, leading directly to the 2:00 PM energy crash.
- A properly constructed gut-healthy bowl always includes a dense base of complex carbohydrates (like quinoa or sweet potatoes) to provide a slow, steady release of energy.
- Commercial bottled salad dressings are often packed with refined oils, sugars, and emulsifiers that actively inflame and damage the delicate lining of your gut.
- Homemade dressings using kefir or yogurt serve as a powerful delivery system, coating your high-fiber lunch in billions of living, beneficial bacteria.
- You must never microwave your live fermented foods; always pack probiotic dressings and krauts in a separate container and add them to your meal only after heating.

Chapter 7: Dinners the Whole Family Will Actually Eat

(Recipes)

It is 5:45 PM on a Wednesday. You just walked through the front door, dropped your bag, and walked into the kitchen. You are exhausted. You look in the fridge and pull out the ingredients for the gut-healing dinner you planned for yourself. You have some wild salmon, a massive pile of Brussels sprouts, and some fermented radishes.

Then you look over at your kids, or maybe your spouse, who is already making a face. They tell you they are absolutely not eating that. They want macaroni and cheese, or maybe ordering a pizza.

So, what do you do? You end up cooking your expensive salmon in one pan, and boiling a box of macaroni in another. You eat your meal feeling isolated, and then you spend the next forty-five minutes washing two completely different sets of dishes.

I get it. It is exhausting. Being a short-order cook for a family that refuses to eat health food is the number one reason people abandon their diets.

This drives me nuts too. We create this artificial wall between what we consider healthy and what we consider comforting. We think a gut-healing dinner has to look like a clinical, unseasoned bowl of raw vegetables, and anything that actually tastes good is bad for us.

Wait — actually, no. That is completely backward.

You can heal your digestion, feed your microbiome, and satisfy a family of four using the exact same pot of food. You just have to learn how to bridge the gap.

Bridging health and comfort

Your gut bacteria do not care if your food looks like a sad diet meal. They only care about the chemical composition of the food you swallow. They want complex carbohydrates, diverse plant fibers, and polyphenols.

You can deliver all of those things wrapped in a meal that looks and tastes like standard Tuesday night comfort food.

The secret is sneaking diverse plants into familiar formats. People resist change when a meal looks unrecognizable. If you put a plate of fermented tempeh and raw seaweed in front of a picky eater, they will reject it immediately. But if you put a massive bowl of spaghetti and meat sauce in front of them, they will devour it.

Our job is to take the spaghetti and meat sauce and quietly upgrade its biological value. We are going to stretch the meat with heavy, prebiotic fibers, hide the vegetables inside the sauce, and use whole grains to anchor the blood sugar. The family gets the comfort food they crave, and your large intestine gets the fertilizer it needs.

The hidden plant strategy

I worked with a mother named Rachel who was on the verge of giving up. She was thirty-eight, dealing with severe irritable bowel syndrome, and had two young boys who would only eat foods that were beige. Chicken nuggets, french fries, and buttered noodles.

Rachel was spending her evenings making two completely separate dinners. She was resentful, tired, and her digestion was actually getting worse because the stress of cooking was shutting down her vagus nerve.

I told Rachel to stop cooking two meals. We were going to hijack the beige food.

I gave her the recipe for the Hidden-Lentil Bolognese. In a standard bolognese, you use ground beef, tomatoes, and some onions. In our version, we use half the amount of ground beef. We replace the other half with cooked brown lentils, finely grated carrots, and minced mushrooms.

When you cook lentils and mushrooms down in a rich tomato sauce, they absorb all the savory flavors of the meat. They physically mimic the texture of ground beef. When Rachel served it over lentil-based pasta, her kids inhaled it. They asked for seconds. They had no idea they just ate three different types of prebiotic fiber, massive amounts of polyphenols from the tomatoes, and highly digestible plant protein.

Rachel only washed one pot. She ate the exact same meal as her kids, her stomach felt great the next morning, and she got her evenings back.

Dinners that do the heavy lifting

The complete cookbook section includes 20 different dinner recipes designed specifically for this purpose. We focus heavily on one-pot and one-pan meals to minimize the dirty dishes. But I want to give you three of the heavy hitters right now.

Hidden-Lentil Bolognese This is the ultimate transition meal. You start by tossing half a pound of ground beef or turkey into a large pot. As it browns, you add half a cup of dried brown lentils, a grated carrot, and a cup of finely chopped mushrooms. You pour in a large jar of crushed tomatoes, a heavy handful of oregano, and let the whole thing simmer for thirty minutes. The lentils break down and become incredibly soft, blending perfectly into the meat. Serve this over chickpea pasta or whole wheat noodles. The resistant starch from the lentils and the fiber from the pasta will keep your digestion moving perfectly the next day.

Gut-Friendly Taco Tuesday Tacos are a fantastic vehicle for dietary diversity. Instead of frying ground beef in cheap vegetable oil, we bake an entire tray of chicken breasts, bell peppers, and red onions. You slice them up for fajita-style tacos. The secret here is the beans. Instead of buying canned refried beans, which are often loaded with inflammatory lard and preservatives, you mash your own black beans with a fork and a splash of chicken broth. Serve the tacos in corn tortillas, which are naturally a whole grain. For the topping, skip the heavy sour cream and use the plain kefir ranch we talked about in the lunch chapter.

One-Pan Mediterranean Chicken and Beans This requires almost zero active cooking time. You take a large baking sheet. You place four chicken thighs on the pan. You open two cans of white cannellini beans, rinse them thoroughly to remove the gas-causing sugars, and pour them around the chicken. Add two cups of cherry tomatoes and a handful of whole garlic cloves. Drizzle the entire pan with olive oil, salt, and rosemary. Bake it at four hundred degrees for forty-five minutes. The tomatoes burst and create a natural sauce. The beans roast in the chicken juices, absorbing massive flavor while providing incredible amounts of soluble fiber. You bring the whole pan to the table, and everyone serves themselves.

Modifying for picky eaters

Now, here is the thing. Even with familiar formats, sometimes you want to add an ingredient that your family simply will not tolerate. Maybe you want to add a giant scoop of sour kimchi to your bowl, or a heavy sprinkle of pumpkin seeds.

The rule here is simple. You cook a baseline meal that everyone accepts, and you modify your own plate at the table.

If you are making the One-Pan Mediterranean Chicken, you bake it exactly as described. When you sit down to eat, you dish out the chicken and beans for your kids. Then, right on your own plate, you stir in a spoonful of raw white miso paste or a pile of fresh sauerkraut.

You are not cooking twice. You are just assembling differently at the very end. This protects your time and your sanity, while still ensuring your microbiome gets exactly what it needs.

Try this now. Pick a meal your family already loves, and figure out how to stretch it with one cheap, high-fiber ingredient.

Action Step: The Bolognese Test

Upgrade your classic pasta night by adding more plant-based fiber without sacrificing the familiar flavor and texture of the dish.

1. The next time you make pasta, buy **half the amount of ground meat** you would normally use.
2. Add **one can of brown lentils** to your shopping list.
3. Rinse the lentils thoroughly before using them.
4. Cook the ground meat as usual. Once it has browned, stir in the rinsed lentils and your tomato sauce.
5. Let the sauce simmer for **20 minutes** so the flavors blend together.
6. Serve the meal to your family without highlighting the ingredient swap. See whether anyone notices the added plant fiber and the subtle change in texture.

Chapter 7 Takeaways

- You do not need to cook separate meals to heal your gut; familiar comfort foods can be easily modified to support a healthy microbiome.
- Sneaking finely chopped vegetables and legumes into sauces, like lentil bolognese, provides massive prebiotic fiber without triggering picky eaters.
- One-pan meals drastically reduce cooking stress and cleanup, which directly lowers the nervous system anxiety that worsens digestion.
- Always build a widely accepted baseline meal for the family, and add your specific fermented foods or raw fibers to your own plate at the table.

- Replacing half the meat in a standard recipe with beans or lentils saves money while dramatically increasing the resistant starch necessary for healthy bowel movements.

Speaking of which, dinner is rarely the end of the story. About two hours after you wash the dishes, you usually find yourself sitting on the couch, staring at the television, feeling a very specific craving. Let's talk about how to handle your sweet tooth without destroying your stomach.

Chapter 8: Microbiome-Friendly Snacks and Sweets

(Recipes)

It is 8:30 PM. The house is finally quiet. You are sitting on the couch watching a show, and suddenly, you want sugar. You don't want a piece of celery. You don't want a glass of water. You want chocolate, or ice cream, or a handful of cookies.

You try to fight it. You tell yourself, "I am trying to heal my gut. Sugar feeds bad bacteria. If I eat a cookie now, I am ruining all the hard work I did today." You white-knuckle your way through the evening, feeling miserable and deprived. Or worse, you give in, eat half a sleeve of cookies, and spend the rest of the night drowning in guilt and physical bloating.

This part gets tricky for almost everyone.

The diet industry has conditioned us to believe that absolute deprivation is the only path to health. They tell us that if we want a happy gut, we must permanently banish all sweets and snacks from our lives.

That is awfulizing. It is a rigid, all-or-nothing mindset that practically guarantees you will eventually binge and fail.

Truth is, deprivation leads directly to diet failure. We all want to feel comforted. We all want to enjoy our food. And the good news is, you can actually use desserts and snacks to actively improve your microbiome. You just have to change the ingredients.

The power of polyphenols

When we think of sweets, we usually think of refined white sugar. Refined sugar is rapidly absorbed in the small intestine. It spikes your blood glucose, and it can feed inflammatory microbes.

But not all sweets are created equal. Let's talk about dark chocolate and berries.

These foods are packed with a specific type of plant compound called *polyphenols*. Polyphenols are essentially antioxidants, but they act very uniquely in the human digestive tract. Most polyphenols are not absorbed in the upper stomach. They travel all the way down to the large intestine, where your good bacteria break them down.

When your bacteria ferment polyphenols, they produce byproducts that reduce inflammation, protect the gut lining, and even lower blood pressure.

Dietary polyphenols significantly modulate the composition of the gut microbiota, acting selectively to inhibit pathogenic bacteria while stimulating the growth of beneficial strains (Cardona et al., 2013).

Dark chocolate—specifically chocolate that is seventy percent cacao or higher—is literal food for your microbiome. Blueberries, raspberries, and blackberries are absolute polyphenol bombs.

When you combine dark chocolate and berries, you are not cheating on your diet. You are deliberately administering medicine to your gut bacteria.

Sweets that do the work

In the book, we have 15 recipes dedicated to snacks and sweets. These are not sad, flavorless diet foods. These are rich, satisfying treats that use complex fibers and whole fruits to satisfy your brain while feeding your stomach.

Dark Chocolate Chia Pudding This is the ultimate evening dessert. You take three tablespoons of chia seeds and put them in a small jar. You add a tablespoon of raw cocoa powder and a tiny drizzle of real maple syrup. You pour in three-quarters of a cup of unsweetened almond milk or kefir. Stir it well, let it sit for five minutes, and stir it again. Put it in the fridge for an hour. The chia seeds absorb the liquid and swell, creating a thick, rich pudding texture. You get the deep comfort of chocolate, but you are consuming nearly ten grams of pure soluble fiber. This fiber slows down the absorption of the maple syrup, preventing a blood sugar spike. You go to bed satisfied, and you wake up with perfect digestion.

Spiced Roasted Chickpeas Sometimes you don't want sweet; you want salty and crunchy. You want a bag of potato chips. Instead, you take a can of chickpeas, rinse them well, and dry them thoroughly with a paper towel. Toss them in olive oil, smoked paprika, garlic powder, and a heavy pinch of salt. Roast them in the oven at four hundred degrees for twenty-five minutes until they are entirely crispy. You get the exact same satisfying crunch as a potato chip, but you are eating dense resistant starch and plant protein.

Berry-Kefir Popsicles If it is summer and you want ice cream, this is the easiest swap. You blend a cup of plain kefir with two cups of frozen mixed berries and half a banana. Pour the thick mixture into cheap plastic popsicle molds and freeze them. You are eating billions of live probiotics wrapped in the sweetness of whole fruit.

Smart snacking versus grazing

Before you start making chia pudding and roasting chickpeas, we need to talk about timing. Because *what* you snack on is important, but *when* you snack dictates whether your gut actually heals.

I see people all the time who eat perfectly healthy food, but they graze all day long. They have a handful of nuts at 10 AM, an apple at 11 AM, half a sandwich at 1 PM, some crackers at 3 PM, and a bowl of popcorn at 9 PM. They never stop eating.

If you graze constantly, you will remain perpetually bloated.

Here is why. Your digestive tract has a built-in cleaning system called the *migrating motor complex*, or the MMC.

Think of the MMC like a street sweeper. About ninety minutes after you finish a meal, your stomach and small intestine initiate a series of strong, sweeping muscular waves. These waves sweep all the leftover food particles, undigested fibers, and lingering bacteria down into the large intestine. It cleans the streets.

But the street sweeper only runs when the road is completely empty of cars.

If you eat a handful of almonds while the MMC is trying to clean, the system immediately shuts down to process the new food (Deloose et al., 2012). If you graze all day, the street sweeper never runs. Old food particles sit in your small intestine and begin to ferment in the wrong place. This leads directly to painful gas, bloating, and a condition known as Small Intestinal Bacterial Overgrowth (SIBO).

You must give your stomach time to rest.

Eat a large, filling breakfast. Then stop eating. Do not eat anything for four hours. Let the street sweeper run. Eat a filling lunch. Stop eating. Let the sweeper run.

If you genuinely need a snack, eat it intentionally. Sit down, put your spiced chickpeas in a bowl, and eat them. Then close the kitchen. Smart snacking is intentional. Mindless grazing is destructive.

Sweetening with whole fruit

When you do make your treats, try to lean on whole fruits for sweetness whenever possible.

If you bake a batch of oat muffins, instead of pouring in half a cup of white sugar, use two overly ripe, mashed bananas. The bananas provide the sweetness your brain wants, but they also bring their structural fiber with them. That fiber acts like a brake pedal on your digestion, slowly releasing the natural sugars into your bloodstream.

You won't master this overnight. Sometimes you are just going to eat a standard piece of cake at a birthday party. From what I've seen, that is completely fine. One piece of cake does not destroy a healthy microbiome, just like one salad does not fix a broken one.

But for your daily habits, you need a reliable alternative that satisfies you without punishing you.

Action Step: The Pudding Swap

Satisfy your chocolate craving with a simple, fiber-rich dessert that you can prepare in just a few minutes.

1. Buy a bag of **whole chia seeds** and some **unsweetened cocoa powder** during your next grocery trip.
2. This evening, instead of reaching for cookies or ice cream, spend a few minutes preparing the **Dark Chocolate Chia Pudding**.
3. Place it in the refrigerator and let it chill while you relax or watch your favorite show.
4. Enjoy it later in the evening and notice how it satisfies your chocolate craving while leaving you feeling comfortably full rather than overly heavy.

Chapter 8 Takeaways

- Strict dietary deprivation usually leads to binge eating; enjoying microbiome-friendly treats is essential for long-term consistency.
- Polyphenols found in dark chocolate and berries act as powerful antioxidants that selectively feed beneficial gut bacteria and reduce internal inflammation.
- The Migrating Motor Complex (MMC) is your gut's internal cleaning system; it only activates when you are fasting between meals.
- Mindless, continuous grazing shuts down the MMC, leaving undigested food in the small intestine which causes severe bloating.

- Using whole fruits like bananas or berries to sweeten snacks provides necessary fiber that slows down the absorption of sugar into the bloodstream.

Funny thing about that pudding, you often need something to wash it down. And we waste a staggering amount of money on drinks that claim to heal us. Let's head to the beverage aisle and look at the reality of expensive tonics, and how to make them at home for pennies.

Chapter 9: Gut-Soothing Tonics and Broths

(Recipes)

You are standing in the checkout line at a trendy grocery store. You feel a little sluggish, so you reach into the refrigerated cooler and grab a glass bottle of commercial kombucha. The label has beautiful, earthy artwork. It promises to deliver billions of living probiotics, detoxify your liver, and heal your gut.

The cashier scans it. It costs five dollars and fifty cents.

You drink it in the car. It tastes sweet, fizzy, and slightly tangy. You feel a little better, mostly because you believe you just did something incredibly healthy for your body.

But let's look at the actual reality of that five-dollar bottle.

The commercial kombucha reality

Kombucha is traditionally a fermented tea. In its pure, home-brewed form, it is quite tart, highly acidic, and packed with diverse yeasts and bacteria.

But traditional kombucha does not sell well to the mass market. It is too sour. So, commercial beverage companies heavily modify it.

To make it taste like soda, they add massive amounts of sugar or fruit juice after the fermentation process is complete. If you look closely at the nutrition label on that bottle, you might find fifteen to twenty grams of added sugar. You are essentially drinking a slightly sour soda.

Even worse, the logistics of shipping living bacteria across the country are incredibly difficult. If a bottle of raw kombucha gets too warm on a delivery truck, the yeast will continue to ferment the sugar, creating carbon dioxide until the glass bottle explodes. To prevent this, many commercial brands pasteurize their kombucha.

We talked about this earlier. Heat kills bacteria. They boil the kombucha to kill the yeast and stabilize the bottle, and then they often artificially inject a single, cheap strain of lab-grown probiotics back into the liquid just so they can legally put the word "probiotic" on the label (Marco et al., 2021).

You just paid five dollars for sugary tea and dead bacteria.

Look, staying hydrated is critical for gut health. We established in the fiber chapter that fiber without water turns into concrete in your intestines. But drinking plain water all day can get boring. You want flavor. You want something warm and soothing in the winter, and something cold and fizzy in the summer.

You can have all of that. You just have to stop buying it in expensive glass bottles.

Making cheap gut drinks at home

We are going to build a routine of gut-soothing tonics and broths that you can make in your own kitchen for pennies. These drinks actually contain the building blocks your digestive tract needs to physically repair itself.

In the recipe section, there are 10 specific drinks designed for this. I want to highlight the three most important ones. They serve different purposes: repairing, soothing, and refreshing.

1. The 24-Hour Bone Broth (The Repair Tool) If your gut is heavily inflamed, or if you suspect you have intestinal permeability (often called leaky gut), this is your primary medicine. When you take animal bones—like leftover chicken carcasses or cheap beef marrow bones—and simmer them in water for a long time, the bones break down. They release massive amounts of collagen, gelatin, and specific amino acids, primarily *L-glutamine*. L-glutamine is the primary fuel source for the cells that line your intestines. Think of it like spackle for a damaged drywall. It physically helps patch the microscopic gaps in your gut lining, reducing inflammation and food sensitivities (Kim & Kim, 2017). You do not need to buy twenty-dollar bags of powdered collagen. You just put a leftover roast chicken carcass in a slow cooker, cover it with water, add a chopped onion and a splash of apple cider vinegar (the acid helps pull the minerals from the bones), and turn it on low for twenty-four hours. Strain the liquid, add some salt, and drink a warm mug of it every morning. It costs almost nothing.

2. Ginger-Mint Tummy Soother Tea (The Relief Tool)
Sometimes your stomach just hurts. Maybe you ate too fast, maybe you are stressed, or maybe you ate a food that disagreed with you. You need immediate, physical relief from the cramping. Commercial teas are fine, but fresh herbs are exponentially stronger. Take a one-inch knob of fresh ginger root. Do not bother peeling it; just slice it thinly. Put the ginger slices and a handful of fresh mint leaves into a mug. Pour boiling water over them, cover the mug with a small plate, and let it steep for ten minutes. Ginger contains compounds called gingerols that actively speed up gastric emptying—meaning they help food move out of your stomach faster, relieving the heavy, bloated feeling. Mint contains menthol, which acts as a natural antispasmodic, physically relaxing the cramping muscles in your intestinal wall. It is fast, cheap, and highly effective.

3. Cheat's Quick Kombucha (The Refresh Tool) If you crave the cold, fizzy, tart experience of a commercial kombucha, but you want to avoid the massive sugar dump and the five-dollar price tag, you make the cheat version. Take a tall glass and fill it with ice. Pour in cold, plain sparkling water. Add one tablespoon of raw, unpasteurized apple cider vinegar. (Make sure the bottle says it contains "the mother"—this is the cloudy web of beneficial bacteria floating at the bottom). Squeeze in the juice of half a lemon. When you stir this up, it hits the exact same flavor notes as a commercial kombucha. It is fizzy, sour, and refreshing. But it contains zero grams of sugar, it costs about twenty cents to make, and the raw apple cider vinegar delivers a legitimate dose of living enzymes and acetic acid, which helps stabilize your blood sugar.

Hydration without the sugar trap

This won't work for everyone instantly. If you are deeply addicted to drinking large amounts of sweet soda or commercial juices, switching to a tart apple cider vinegar drink will shock your palate at first.

You have to awfulize less. Do not tell yourself, "I hate this, I can never drink soda again, my life is ruined." Just start small.

If you normally drink two cans of soda a day, just replace one of them with the Cheat's Kombucha. If you normally buy a sweet coffee drink every afternoon, replace it with the Ginger-Mint tea twice a week.

As your microbiome shifts, your physical cravings will shift. The bad bacteria in your gut that thrive on massive amounts of refined sugar will begin to die off. As they die, they stop sending chemical signals to your brain demanding more sugar. Within a few weeks, that five-dollar bottle of commercial kombucha will actually taste sickeningly sweet to you.

Your palate adapts when your internal garden changes.

Action Step: The Tonic Swap
Replace your usual sugary or expensive drink with a simple homemade alternative that delivers a refreshing, tangy flavor.

1. Identify the drink you reach for most often during the week—such as a commercial kombucha, soda, sweetened iced tea, or another sugary beverage.
2. Pick up a bottle of **raw apple cider vinegar** (with "the mother"), a few lemons, and a box of plain sparkling water during your next grocery trip.
3. The next time you crave your usual afternoon drink, make a **Cheat's Quick Kombucha** instead.

4. Serve it cold and notice how its crisp, tart flavor can satisfy your craving while helping you cut back on added sugar and unnecessary spending.

Chapter 9 Takeaways

- Many expensive commercial kombuchas are pasteurized to prevent explosion during shipping, effectively killing the beneficial bacteria and leaving you with a high-sugar soda.
- Simmering animal bones creates a cheap, highly bioavailable broth packed with L-glutamine, an amino acid that physically repairs the intestinal lining.
- Fresh ginger and mint steeped in hot water provide immediate, physical relief from stomach cramping by accelerating gastric emptying and relaxing intestinal muscles.
- Raw apple cider vinegar mixed with sparkling water perfectly mimics the fizzy, tart experience of kombucha for pennies, without any added sugar.
- As you reduce liquid sugars and increase diverse plant intake, your gut bacteria will shift, naturally reducing your physical cravings for intensely sweet drinks.

Chapter 10: Troubleshooting: The "Flare-Up" Rescue Protocol

You wake up at three in the morning. Your stomach is cramping so hard you have to curl your knees to your chest. You run to the bathroom, sweating, and spend the next hour in absolute misery.

By sunrise, you feel completely drained. Your abdomen is swollen, tender to the touch, and making loud gurgling noises.

Your mind immediately starts racing. You think, "I ruined it. I was doing so well with my new diet, and now my stomach is completely broken again. I must have eaten something toxic. I am never going to heal. This is hopeless."

I get it. It is exhausting to feel like you are back at square one. When you are in physical pain, it is incredibly easy to awfulize the situation. You take a temporary setback and blow it up into a permanent catastrophe.

Truth is, you did not ruin anything. Your body is just reacting to a threat. You are having a gut flare-up.

A flare-up happens to everyone. Maybe you picked up a mild stomach bug from your kid's school. Maybe you ate some undercooked chicken at a barbecue. Maybe you were prescribed a harsh course of antibiotics for a sinus infection, or maybe you just experienced a massive spike in stress at work.

Whatever the trigger, your internal garden is currently on fire. The rules change when there is a fire. If you try to eat your normal, healthy diet today, you are going to make the fire much worse.

Recognizing the signs of a gut flare-up

First, we need to define what an actual flare-up is, versus just a slightly gassy afternoon.

A bit of bloating after a big meal of beans is normal. That is just fermentation. A true flare-up is an inflammatory response in your digestive tract. Your body is trying to expel something, or the mucosal lining of your intestines has become inflamed and irritated.

You know you are in a flare-up if you experience sudden, severe diarrhea, or its complete opposite, a sudden and painful impaction of constipation lasting several days. You might feel sharp, stabbing cramps in your lower abdomen. You will likely lose your appetite entirely, and you might feel nauseous or feverish.

When this happens, your gut bacteria are completely thrown out of balance. The bad bacteria might be temporarily overrunning the good bacteria, and the physical walls of your intestines are highly sensitive.

Why you must temporarily reduce fiber

This is where people make a massive, painful mistake.

I had a client named Greg. Greg went on a vacation to Mexico and got a severe case of food poisoning. For two days, he could barely leave his hotel room. When he finally flew home, he was determined to "fix" his gut immediately.

He told himself, "Fiber is good for the gut. I need to eat as much healthy food as possible to heal."

So, Greg went to the store, bought a massive bag of raw kale, two cans of chickpeas, and some raw broccoli. He made a giant salad and forced himself to eat it, thinking it was medicine.

An hour later, he was in agony. His stomach cramped so violently he almost went to the emergency room.

He didn't understand what went wrong. He ate healthy food. Why was he in pain?

Here is the thing. When your intestinal lining is inflamed from a stomach bug, a flare-up, or food poisoning, it is physically swollen. It is raw.

Think of it like getting a terrible sunburn on your arm. Under normal circumstances, rubbing a rough towel on your arm feels fine. It might even feel like a nice massage. But if you rub that same rough towel over a fresh, blistering sunburn, it is going to cause excruciating pain.

Fiber is the rough towel.

When you are healthy, rough, insoluble fiber is fantastic. It sweeps your intestines clean. But when your intestines are inflamed, that same rough fiber scrapes against the raw, swollen tissue. It causes intense cramping, rapid motility, and severe pain.

During a flare-up, you have to stop eating raw vegetables. You have to stop eating beans. You have to temporarily stop feeding the bacteria, and start resting the tissue.

The 3-day gut rest protocol

When the fire starts, we shift to a *low-residue diet.*

A low-residue diet is exactly what it sounds like. We are choosing foods that leave almost zero residue in your digestive tract. These foods require almost no work from your stomach, and they do not ferment in your large intestine. They give your system a complete break.

You only do this for three days. It is a temporary rescue plan, not a long-term lifestyle.

For these three days, you are going to eat the most boring, easily digestible foods on the planet.

First, the carbohydrates. You drop the complex, heavy grains. You switch to plain white rice, white potatoes without the skin, and plain sourdough toast. White rice is pure, simple starch. It absorbs water in your gut, which helps solidify loose stools if you are dealing with diarrhea, and it digests high up in your system, leaving your lower colon entirely alone.

Second, the proteins. No heavy red meat, no beans, and no fried food. You want plain, boiled or baked chicken breast, or very soft scrambled eggs. These proteins break down effortlessly in your stomach acid.

Third, the liquids. This is where you pull out the 24-Hour Bone Broth we talked about in Chapter 9. The L-glutamine in the bone broth will immediately start patching up the irritated lining of your intestines. Drink warm broth with every single meal.

For three days, Greg's plate should have been a scoop of soft white rice, a piece of plain baked chicken, and a mug of warm bone broth.

It is boring. It is bland. But it stops the cramping almost immediately.

Rebuilding after antibiotics

Quick side note, because this happens frequently. Sometimes you get strep throat or a severe infection, and your doctor prescribes antibiotics.

Take the medicine. Do not awfulize the antibiotics and refuse necessary medical treatment just because you are worried about your microbiome.

But you do need to understand what the medicine does. Antibiotics are like a forest fire. They do not discriminate. They kill the bad bacteria causing your sinus infection, but they also kill a massive portion of the good bacteria in your internal garden.

After you finish a course of antibiotics, your gut is barren. This is why many people experience severe diarrhea during or immediately after taking them.

Broad-spectrum antibiotics cause rapid and significant drops in microbial diversity, shifting the gut environment to a state that is highly susceptible to opportunistic pathogens (Dethlefsen et al., 2008).

You have to rebuild the soil. But you do it slowly.

Do not take your last antibiotic pill and immediately eat a giant bowl of raw cabbage. Your bacteria are gone; there is no one there to ferment the cabbage. It will just sit there and rot, causing massive gas.

Instead, use the 3-Day Gut Rest protocol immediately after your last pill. Give the tissue time to calm down.

Then, on day four, start introducing cooked, soft fibers. Steamed carrots. Roasted sweet potatoes. Small amounts of kefir.

Over the next two weeks, slowly scale your fiber back up using the protocol from Chapter 3. Treat your gut like it is brand new, because chemically, it is. It takes time for the microbial populations to re-establish themselves. Be patient.

When to actually see a gastroenterologist

This part gets tricky. I am giving you nutritional strategies, but I am not your doctor. Food is powerful, but it cannot fix acute medical emergencies.

We try to handle everything ourselves, but sometimes, a flare-up is not just a passing bug. Sometimes it is a sign of a serious, structural medical issue.

You need to know the red flags. If you experience any of these symptoms, you stop trying to fix it with white rice and bone broth, and you call a gastroenterologist immediately.

First: Blood in the toilet. If you see bright red blood, or if your stool looks black and tarry like coffee grounds, that is a sign of internal bleeding. Do not ignore it.

Second: Unexplained, rapid weight loss. If you lose ten pounds in a month without trying, your body is failing to absorb nutrients, or something else is severely wrong.

Third: Extreme, localized pain that does not move. Gas pain moves around your abdomen. If you have a sharp, stabbing pain in one specific spot—especially the lower right side—that could be appendicitis or a severe blockage.

Fourth: A flare-up that lasts longer than two weeks. Food poisoning resolves in a few days. If you are having severe diarrhea for fourteen days straight, you need medical testing to rule out parasitic infections, Crohn's disease, or Ulcerative Colitis.

Do not let fear stop you from getting medical help. Getting a colonoscopy is not a failure of your diet. It is just gathering data.

The mental game of a flare up

When you are in the middle of a bad stomach week, the mental game is harder than the physical game.

You will feel tired. You will feel bloated. You will look in the mirror and hate how your stomach looks.

You have to catch your irrational thoughts. Tell yourself the truth: "My stomach hurts right now, and that is highly inconvenient and uncomfortable, but it is not the end of the world. It will pass. I have a plan."

You switch to the bland food. You drink the broth. You rest on the couch with a heating pad. You give your body the grace it needs to repair the damage.

Action Step: The Rescue Bookmark

Prepare a simple "emergency plan" you can refer to when your digestion feels unsettled.

1. Take a piece of paper or open a note on your phone.
2. Title it: **"The 3-Day Gut Rest"**
3. Add this grocery list:
    - White rice
    - Plain chicken breasts
    - Eggs
    - Sourdough bread
    - Ingredients for bone broth
4. Write this reminder:

"NO raw vegetables, NO beans, NO nuts, NO heavy spices."

5. Save the note somewhere easy to find. The next time you experience a stomach bug or a digestive flare-up, use this prepared plan as a simple guide instead of having to make decisions while you feel unwell.

Section Takeaways

- A gut flare-up is a state of active inflammation; your intestinal walls are physically swollen and highly sensitive.
- Eating heavy, rough fiber during a flare-up acts like sandpaper on a sunburn, dramatically worsening your cramps and pain.
- The 3-Day Gut Rest protocol relies on low-residue foods like white rice and plain chicken that digest quickly without fermenting in the lower colon.

- Antibiotics completely wipe out your gut bacteria; you must rebuild your diet very slowly afterward, starting with soft, cooked vegetables rather than raw salads.
- Never ignore medical red flags like blood in your stool, severe localized pain, or rapid weight loss; these require immediate intervention from a gastroenterologist.

Speaking of which, flare-ups often happen when we leave the safety of our own kitchens. The real test of your new habits is not what you do alone in your house. The real test is what happens when you go out into the world. Let's talk about restaurants, vacations, and staying sane.

Chapter 11: Real World Gut Health

(Dining Out and Travel)

You are sitting at a beautifully lit table in an Italian restaurant. Your friends are laughing, drinking wine, and passing around a massive basket of warm garlic bread. The waiter hands you a menu.

Instead of feeling excited, your chest tightens. Your heart rate speeds up. You stare at the menu, but all you see are threats.

You think, "The pasta has refined flour. The sauce probably has cheap vegetable oil. I don't see any prebiotic fibers on this list. If I eat this food, I am going to ruin my microbiome. I am going to be bloated for a week."

When the waiter comes to you, you panic. You order a plain, dry garden salad with no dressing, and a piece of unseasoned grilled chicken. You sit there, chewing on dry lettuce, feeling entirely isolated while your friends enjoy their evening.

I see this happen constantly. People get so obsessed with healing their digestion that they develop orthorexia—an unhealthy obsession with eating healthy food. They become terrified of restaurants. They stop traveling. They stop going to dinner parties.

This drives me nuts. If your diet forces you to live in a miserable, isolated bubble, then your diet is a failure.

The biology of dining out stress

Here is the most ironic part of that Italian restaurant scenario. Your panic attack at the table did more damage to your digestion than a plate of pasta ever could.

We talked about the vagus nerve in the first chapter. It connects your brain directly to your stomach. When you sit at a restaurant and awfulize the menu, telling yourself that the food is toxic and dangerous, your brain triggers a fight-or-flight response.

Your nervous system pumps out cortisol and adrenaline. Your body thinks it is being chased by a predator. And what does a body do when it is running for its life? It completely shuts down digestion.

Blood flow is diverted away from your stomach and into your muscles. Your stomach acid production drops. Your digestive enzymes stop flowing.

Psychological stress significantly delays gastric emptying and alters intestinal transit, transforming normally digestible meals into triggers for severe functional dyspepsia and bloating (Tache et al., 2001).

If you eat a meal—even a perfectly healthy meal—while in a state of high stress, it will sit in your stomach like a rock. It will ferment poorly, and you will get bloated.

If you want to digest restaurant food properly, you have to relax. You have to accept that one imperfect meal does not destroy a healthy microbiome. Your internal garden is resilient. It can handle a plate of pasta on a Friday night, as long as you feed it properly on Saturday morning.

Navigating the standard menu

That being said, you don't have to completely abandon your habits when you eat out. You just have to learn how to navigate the menu quietly and effectively.

Most restaurants, even standard chain restaurants, have gut-friendly options if you know how to look for them. We are looking for "stealth veggies" and complex proteins.

Let's look at a classic American steakhouse or grill.

Instead of ordering the massive burger with a mountain of deep-fried potatoes, look at the sides. Most grills offer baked potatoes, roasted Brussels sprouts, or grilled asparagus.

Order a modest steak or a piece of grilled salmon. Ask for a baked potato. Here is the trick: eat the skin of the baked potato. The skin contains massive amounts of dense fiber. Ask them to swap the french fries for a side of roasted broccoli.

You just built a meal that contains high-quality protein, resistant starch, and cruciferous vegetables. It is a fantastic gut-healthy meal, and you didn't have to be the weird person ordering dry lettuce.

If you are at a Mexican restaurant, you are actually in luck. Mexican cuisine is inherently gut-friendly if you avoid the deep fryer. Fajitas are incredible. You get a massive sizzling plate of onions and bell peppers (huge prebiotic fibers). You get grilled chicken or steak. Ask for a side of black beans instead of the refried beans. Skip the massive flour tortillas and ask for soft corn tortillas instead, which are a whole grain.

You eat a massive, flavorful meal, and your gut bacteria get a feast.

The fast food survival guide

Sometimes, you don't have the luxury of a sit-down restaurant. You are driving down the highway, you have ten minutes, and your only options are fast food drive-thrus.

Do not panic. You can survive this without a massive flare-up.

The biggest issue with fast food is the refined seed oils used in the deep fryers. These oils are highly inflammatory to the gut lining. Your first rule at a fast food place is simple: Do not order anything fried. No fries, no crispy chicken, no hash browns.

If you are at a standard burger place, order a double burger, but ask for it wrapped in lettuce instead of the heavily processed bun. The bun is just cheap, sugary starch that will spike your blood sugar and feed bad bacteria. The meat, lettuce, and tomatoes will digest cleanly.

If you can find a bowl-based chain, like Chipotle or Cava, you have hit the jackpot. These are fast-food goldmines for your microbiome.

At a burrito bowl place, you can build a masterpiece. Ask for brown rice, black beans, fajita vegetables, chicken, and a massive scoop of pico de gallo and guacamole. You are getting close to ten different plant types, complex fibers, and healthy fats in a single, cheap, fast bowl.

Travel and the time zone effect

Now, let's talk about travel.

I have clients who eat perfectly at home, but the second they step onto an airplane, their digestion completely stops. They go on a five-day vacation and do not use the bathroom once. They spend the whole trip feeling heavy and miserable.

There are two reasons this happens.

First, dehydration. Airplane cabins have extremely low humidity. You lose a massive amount of water just by breathing recycled air. As we know, fiber without water equals concrete. If you eat your normal high-fiber snacks on a plane but don't drink double your normal amount of water, you will become severely constipated.

Second, jet lag.

Your gut bacteria actually have their own circadian rhythm. They know when it is day, and they know when it is night. They expect food during the day, and they expect to rest and clean the intestines at night.

When you fly across three time zones, you confuse your bacteria. You land, and you eat a massive dinner at 8:00 PM local time. But your gut bacteria think it is 2:00 AM. They are asleep. They are not producing the necessary enzymes to break down the food.

Disruption of the circadian clock through travel or shift work directly alters the composition and function of the gut microbiome, leading to metabolic and digestive disturbances (Thaiss et al., 2014).

Here is the travel hack to fix this. When you are flying across multiple time zones, try to fast during the flight. Drink massive amounts of water, but do not eat the heavy airplane food.

Wait until you land. When you arrive at your destination, eat your first meal at the normal local mealtime. This sends a loud biological signal to your gut bacteria, essentially resetting their clocks to the new time zone.

Alcohol and the microbiome

We have to talk about alcohol. People always ask, "Do I have to quit drinking entirely to have a healthy gut?"

Truth is, alcohol is a toxin. It irritates the gut lining, and heavy drinking will destroy your microbiome. But you do not have to become a strict teetotaler if you enjoy a drink with friends. You just have to be smart about what you order.

The worst things you can drink are heavy, sugary cocktails. Margaritas made from cheap syrups, rum and colas, or sweet daiquiris. The combination of alcohol and massive amounts of refined sugar feeds yeast overgrowths in your gut and causes immediate inflammation.

Beer is tricky. It contains gluten and heavy carbohydrates. Many people find that beer causes severe, immediate bloating.

If you are going to drink, stick to the cleaner options.

A glass of dry red wine is actually beneficial in small amounts. Red wine is packed with polyphenols from the grape skins, which, as we learned in Chapter 8, feed the good bacteria.

If you don't like wine, stick to clear liquors. A vodka with plain soda water and a squeeze of fresh lime contains zero sugar and will not trigger a massive inflammatory response in your lower intestines.

Drink one glass of water for every alcoholic drink you consume. It dilutes the alcohol in your stomach and protects your mucosal lining.

You can live a normal life. You can go to parties. You can eat at restaurants. You just have to make slightly better choices, and most importantly, you have to stop stressing out over the menu.

Action Step: The Menu Rehearsal

Make healthy restaurant choices easier by planning ahead before you arrive.

1. Think of the restaurant your family or friends visit most often.
2. Go online and look up the menu before your next visit.
3. Without the pressure of making a quick decision at the table, find **two meals** that fit your gut-friendly framework:
    - Include a quality protein source
    - Include vegetables where possible
    - Avoid heavily deep-fried options
4. Write down your two choices so you have them ready.
5. The next time you visit that restaurant, you can order with confidence without needing to study the menu or make a big change to your usual routine.

Chapter 11 Takeaways

- High stress and anxiety over finding the "perfect" meal at a restaurant shuts down your vagus nerve, halting digestion and guaranteeing you will be bloated regardless of what you eat.

- Standard chain restaurants offer great gut-friendly options if you swap deep-fried sides for roasted vegetables or baked potatoes (eating the skin for fiber).
- When eating fast food, avoid refined seed oils by skipping all fried items; opt for bowl-based meals with rice, beans, and fresh salsas.
- Air travel dehydrates the body and disrupts the circadian rhythm of your gut bacteria, leading to severe travel constipation; fasting on the plane and hydrating heavily prevents this.
- If consuming alcohol, avoid high-sugar cocktails and heavy beers; opt for dry red wine, which provides beneficial polyphenols, or clear liquors with plain soda water.

Before I forget, once you start living this way, you are going to want proof. You are going to want to know if all this cabbage and oat-eating is actually changing anything inside you. Let's talk about how to measure your success without getting scammed by the medical testing industry.

Chapter 12: Tracking Success

(Without $200 Stool Tests)

You are scrolling through your phone on the couch, and an ad pops up. It is a sleek, modern video featuring a doctor in a white coat. He tells you that you cannot possibly know what is wrong with your gut unless you take his company's proprietary microbiome test.

For just two hundred and fifty dollars, they will send you a plastic tube. You put a sample of your stool in the tube, mail it to their lab, and they will send you a beautiful, color-coded report detailing every single strain of bacteria in your body.

You think, "This is it. This is the missing piece. If I just get the data, I will finally know how to eat."

You pull out your credit card and buy the kit. A month later, you get the report. It is a massive spreadsheet listing hundreds of unpronounceable bacterial names. It says your *Firmicutes* are slightly high and your *Bacteroidetes* are slightly low.

You stare at it, completely confused. What does that actually mean? Do you eat more beans? Less chicken? The report doesn't really tell you. It just suggests you buy their specific, expensive probiotic blends to fix the numbers.

I see this constantly. People want hard data to prove their diet is working, so they waste hundreds of dollars on commercial stool tests.

The reality of commercial testing

Here is the dirty secret of the commercial microbiome testing industry. Right now, the science is simply not advanced enough to give you actionable, personalized dietary advice based on a single stool sample.

Your microbiome is not static. It is highly dynamic.

If you eat a massive bowl of broccoli on Tuesday, and take a stool test on Wednesday, your results will show a massive spike in fiber-loving bacteria. If you eat a steak and drink two beers on Friday, and take a test on Saturday, your results will look completely different.

Commercial microbiome tests currently lack the clinical validation required to accurately predict disease risk or prescribe highly specific dietary interventions, as microbial populations fluctuate wildly based on daily transit and short-term diet (Bashiardes et al., 2016).

You are paying two hundred dollars for a snapshot of what you ate two days ago. It does not give you a permanent map of your health.

You do not need a laboratory to tell you if your internal garden is thriving. Your body gives you free, incredibly accurate bio-feedback every single day. You just have to know how to read the signals.

The Bristol Stool Chart

This part gets tricky for some people, because we are conditioned to be embarrassed about our bodily functions. We go to the bathroom, flush as quickly as possible, and never look in the toilet bowl.

That is a massive mistake. Your stool is the daily report card of your digestive system.

Gastroenterologists use a clinical tool called the Bristol Stool Chart. It categorizes human waste into seven distinct types. Once you understand this chart, you will know exactly how much fiber and water you need for the day.

Let's break down the seven types.

Type 1: Separate hard lumps, like nuts. This is severe constipation. Your transit time is way too slow. The stool has been sitting in your large intestine for days, and your body has absorbed all the water out of it. You are likely highly dehydrated and severely lacking in soluble fiber (like oats and beans).

Type 2: Sausage-shaped, but lumpy. Mild constipation. You are getting closer, but you still need more water and likely more movement to stimulate the migrating motor complex.

Type 3: Like a sausage but with cracks on its surface. This is considered normal and healthy. You are doing well.

Type 4: Like a sausage or snake, smooth and soft. This is the holy grail of digestion. This is what you are aiming for. A smooth, cohesive stool means you have the perfect balance of rough insoluble fiber to give it bulk, soluble fiber to make it soft, and adequate hydration. When you consistently produce Type 4, your microbiome is thriving.

Type 5: Soft blobs with clear-cut edges. This is slightly loose. It often happens if you suddenly increase your fiber intake too quickly, or if you eat a meal heavily loaded with fats that your liver struggled to break down.

Type 6: Fluffy pieces with ragged edges, a mushy stool. Mild diarrhea. Your transit time is too fast. Your large intestine did not have time to extract the water. This can be caused by food sensitivities, a mild flare-up, or high stress.

Type 7: Watery, no solid pieces. Severe diarrhea. This is the hallmark of a severe stomach bug, food poisoning, or an extreme inflammatory flare-up. Switch immediately to the 3-Day Gut Rest protocol.

You do not need a lab test. If you look in the toilet and see Type 1, you know you need to drink two massive glasses of water and eat some oatmeal. If you see Type 4, you know exactly what you did yesterday worked, and you should keep doing it.

Tracking the non-scale victories

Digestion is not just about the bathroom. As your microbiome heals, it stops sending distress signals up the vagus nerve. You will notice profound changes in the rest of your body.

I tell my clients to track three specific things when they start this diet.

First, track your 2:00 PM energy. Before you started eating gut-healthy bowls for lunch, you probably needed a double espresso just to keep your eyes open in the afternoon. When your microbiome is fed properly with complex carbohydrates, that afternoon crash vanishes. Waking up feeling rested and surviving the afternoon without caffeine is a massive sign of gut healing.

Second, look at your skin. Your skin and your gut are closely linked through the immune system. Chronic skin conditions like eczema, rosacea, and adult acne are often driven by systemic inflammation originating in an unhappy large intestine. As you increase your dietary diversity and lower your reliance on highly processed foods, you will often find your skin clears up dramatically.

Third, track your brain fog. When your gut bacteria ferment heavy sugars and refined foods in the wrong place, they can produce byproducts like D-lactic acid, which literally causes a feeling of intoxication and mental fog. When you eat clean, peasant foods, that fog lifts. You can focus on a spreadsheet for an hour without losing your train of thought.

These are the real metrics of success.

The transit time test

If you want a fun, entirely free scientific experiment to see how your gut is functioning, you can run the Transit Time Test.

Transit time is the amount of time it takes for food to enter your mouth and exit your body. A healthy transit time is usually between twenty-four and thirty-six hours.

If your transit time is seventy-two hours, you have severe sluggishness, and bad bacteria are likely fermenting old food, causing bloating. If your transit time is twelve hours, your body is rushing food through so quickly that you are not absorbing your nutrients.

To test this, you use a marker food. You need a food that passes through you visibly unchanged.

The easiest options are sweet corn or red beets.

Here is how you do it. Pick a day, let's say Saturday morning at 9:00 AM. Eat a massive spoonful of whole kernel corn, or eat a small bowl of roasted red beets. Write down the exact time you ate it.

Then, you wait. Over the next few days, you check the toilet.

Because humans cannot fully digest the outer hull of a corn kernel, you will see it clearly in your stool. If you used beets, your stool (and possibly your urine) will turn a bright, unmistakable red-purple color.

When you see the marker in the toilet, write down the time. Calculate the hours between eating the marker and seeing the marker.

If it took twenty-eight hours, you have a beautifully functioning, efficient digestive tract. You have proof, right there in your own bathroom, that your internal engine is running perfectly.

Celebrating the reality

Healing your gut is not about reaching a state of absolute medical perfection. It is not about taking a test and getting a perfect score.

It is about getting your life back.

It is about putting on a pair of jeans at 8:00 AM and knowing they will still fit comfortably at 8:00 PM because you are not going to inflate like a balloon.

It is about going to a restaurant with your family and actually enjoying the conversation, rather than quietly panicking over the menu.

It is about walking down the supplement aisle at the grocery store, looking at the fifty-dollar probiotic pills and the eighty-dollar greens powders, and walking right past them. You do not need them anymore. You have a cutting board, a sharp knife, and a kitchen full of cheap, powerful, real food.

You have everything you need.

Action Step: The Beet Test

Use a natural food marker to estimate how long it takes food to move through your digestive system.

1. Buy a bunch of **fresh red beets** or a can of **whole-kernel corn**.
2. Choose a specific time the next day to eat a generous serving of your chosen marker food (for example, lunch at **12:00 PM**).
3. Write down the exact **date and time** you ate the marker food and place the note somewhere visible, such as your bathroom mirror.
4. Pay attention to your bowel movements over the next **three days**.
5. When you notice the marker—such as the red pigment from beets or visible corn kernels—calculate your estimated transit time from when you ate the food to when you observed the marker.

6. Use this information as a guide for adjusting your water and fiber habits, with the goal of supporting a comfortable, consistent transit time.

Final Thoughts

- Commercial microbiome stool tests are currently a waste of money for the average person, as microbial populations shift daily based on short-term diet, rendering the reports highly inaccurate over time.
- The Bristol Stool Chart is a free, clinically accurate tool; consistently producing Type 4 (smooth, soft, snake-like) stools is the ultimate proof of a healthy microbiome.
- Physical energy levels, the clearance of brain fog, and the reduction of skin inflammation are powerful, non-scale indicators that your gut lining is healing.
- Measuring your personal transit time using corn or beets allows you to diagnose whether your digestive tract is sluggish (causing bloat) or hyperactive (causing nutrient malabsorption).
- True digestive success is measured by the absence of pain, the ability to eat socially without fear, and the financial freedom of no longer relying on expensive supplements.

Conclusion: Trust Your Gut

(And Your Grocery Store)

You are walking through the sliding glass doors of your local supermarket. It is a Tuesday evening. You grab a shopping cart and start making your way down the familiar aisles. You pick up a heavy head of green cabbage, a bag of dried black beans, some plain rolled oats, and a carton of kefir. You throw some garlic, onions, and sweet potatoes into the cart.

Then, you turn the corner and find yourself standing at the end of the health and wellness aisle.

You stop for a second and look down the row. You see the glowing plastic bottles lined up perfectly on the shelves. You see the fifty-dollar tubs of green powder claiming to fix your digestion. You see the refrigerated case full of expensive, specialized probiotic capsules. You see the gummies, the detox teas, and the digestive enzymes.

A few months ago, you would have stopped here. You would have spent twenty minutes reading the tiny print on the back of those bottles, feeling a tight knot of anxiety in your chest. You would have worried that if you did not buy the right pill, your stomach would never stop hurting. You would have swiped your credit card, spending money you actually needed for other things, just to buy a temporary sense of hope.

But today? You just look at the shelves, shake your head slightly, and keep pushing your cart right past them.

You do not need anything down that aisle. You already have everything your body requires sitting right there in the basket of your cart. It cost you about fifteen dollars, and it is going to work better than any isolated chemical powder ever could.

That specific moment—the moment you realize you are entirely capable of managing your own physical health using ordinary, everyday food—is the ultimate goal of this entire process. You are no longer dependent on an industry that profits from your confusion. You have taken your power back, right there in the produce section.

Between us, getting to this point is not easy. I know exactly how hard you have worked to change your daily habits. But as we wrap up our time together, we need to address the final psychological hurdle that trips up almost everyone.

The fear of falling off the wagon

You have read the science. You have cleared out your pantry, survived the four-week fiber protocol, and learned how to sneak fermented foods into your dinners. You are finally experiencing days without painful bloating. You have energy at two in the afternoon.

But in the back of your mind, there is a nagging, persistent fear.

You find yourself lying in bed at night, caught in a 3 AM worry spiral. You think, "What if I mess this up? What if I go to a party this weekend and eat a bunch of junk food? I will ruin all my progress. My gut bacteria will die, the bloating will come back, and I will be right back where I started. I must never slip up."

This is a massive mental trap.

When we finally find relief from physical pain, we become terrified of losing it. We start making rigid, absolute demands on ourselves. We tell ourselves that we *must* eat perfectly clean at all times, and that any deviation is a total disaster. We awfulize the idea of eating a standard piece of birthday cake or ordering a pizza on a Friday night.

Let's stop right here and look at this belief, because it is entirely irrational.

Perfection is not a biological requirement. Your digestive system is not a fragile house of cards that collapses the second the wind blows.

Think about a massive, healthy forest. A thriving ecosystem is full of diverse plants, strong trees, and millions of living organisms. If someone walks through that forest and drops a single candy wrapper on the ground, does the entire forest suddenly wither and die? Of course not. The forest is robust. It absorbs the minor insult and keeps thriving because its foundation is strong.

Your microbiome works the exact same way.

When you spend months feeding your gut bacteria a massive diversity of plant fibers, complex carbohydrates, and polyphenols, you build a thick, resilient mucosal lining. You build a strong, diverse bacterial workforce.

If you take that strong workforce and throw a greasy cheeseburger and a couple of beers at it on a Saturday night, it is not going to permanently shut down. You might feel slightly sluggish the next morning. You might experience a little bit of temporary gas. But your good bacteria do not instantly vanish.

Long-term dietary patterns establish stable, resilient microbial enterotypes that are capable of withstanding short-term dietary deviations without suffering permanent structural changes (Wu et al., 2011).

Consistency always beats perfection. If you eat thirty different plants a week, prioritize fiber, and hydrate well for eighty percent of your meals, your gut can easily handle whatever you throw at it for the other twenty percent.

You do not need to demand absolute compliance from yourself. The stress and anxiety generated by trying to be a perfect eater will do far more damage to your digestion than a single slice of cake ever could.

Letting go of the patient identity

To truly trust your gut, you have to let go of the idea that you are a permanent patient.

The wellness industry survives by convincing you that you are fundamentally broken. They tell you that your body is constantly under attack from "toxins" and that you are incapable of digesting modern food without their proprietary blends. They assign you the identity of a sick person who requires constant medical management through over-the-counter supplements.

I worked with a woman named Claire who struggled deeply with this. Claire had successfully implemented every single recipe in this book. Her bloating was gone. Her bowel movements were a perfect Type 4 on the Bristol Stool Chart. She felt fantastic.

But she was still taking a sixty-dollar probiotic pill every morning.

I asked her why she was still buying it. She looked at me and said, "I am terrified to stop. What if my stomach breaks again? I know I am eating well, but I just feel like I need the pill as a safety net."

Claire had tied her sense of safety to a plastic bottle instead of trusting her own body. She still viewed herself as a patient.

I challenged her to run an experiment. I told her to put the bottle of probiotics in the back of her closet for two weeks. Just fourteen days. If her stomach completely fell apart, she could go right back to taking them. But she had to rely solely on her food—the kefir, the miso, the oats, the beans—for two weeks.

The first three days, she was highly anxious. She hyper-fixated on every tiny rumble in her stomach, convinced it was the beginning of a massive flare-up.

But by day seven, she noticed something interesting. Nothing had changed. Her digestion was still perfectly fine. By day fourteen, she felt completely normal.

She took the half-empty bottle of expensive probiotics out of her closet and threw it in the trash.

Claire finally realized that the pill was not doing the heavy lifting. The massive bowl of lentil bolognese she cooked for dinner was doing the heavy lifting. The daily chia pudding was doing the work. The apple cider vinegar tonics were keeping things moving.

When you accept that real food is the ultimate medicine, you stop viewing yourself as a fragile patient. You become the active owner of your own health. You are just a person who knows how to feed themselves properly.

The reality of the food matrix

Let's do a quick review of why that grocery store cart works so much better than the supplement aisle. It comes back to the core biological truth we discussed in the very beginning: the food matrix.

We humans are arrogant. We think we can outsmart millions of years of evolution by isolating a single vitamin in a laboratory, drying it out, and putting it in a gelatin capsule.

But your digestive tract is highly intelligent. It evolved to break down complex physical structures. It expects fiber. It expects water. It expects the slow, mechanical process of chewing, followed by the slow, chemical process of acid breakdown.

When you eat a baked potato with the skin on, you are not just getting a dose of potassium. You are getting resistant starch that survives the stomach acid. You are getting physical bulk that sweeps the intestines clean. You are delivering food all the way down to the lowest parts of your colon, right where the bacteria live.

When you swallow a pill, you bypass this entire mechanical process. You dump naked, isolated chemicals into a burning pool of stomach acid. Most of it is destroyed. The rest is absorbed too quickly, spiking your bloodstream and leaving your lower intestine completely starved of the physical material it needs to function.

You cannot cheat the system. You have to do the mechanical work of digesting real food.

Once you understand this, walking past the supplement aisle isn't a sacrifice. It isn't a restriction. It is just common sense. Why would you pay premium prices for a product that biologically bypasses the exact organs you are trying to heal?

The financial relief of real food

This brings me to the money. We need to talk about the financial reality of what you have accomplished.

When we started this process, I asked you to do a Supplement Audit. I asked you to tally up exactly how much money you were spending every month on greens powders, probiotics, gummies, and specialized health drinks.

For the average person struggling with gut issues, that number is usually around one hundred and fifty dollars a month. Sometimes it is much higher.

Let's look at the math. One hundred and fifty dollars a month is one thousand, eight hundred dollars a year.

Over five years, that is nine thousand dollars.

Nine thousand dollars handed over to an industry that largely fails to provide permanent relief, because it treats the symptom instead of feeding the underlying ecosystem.

Now, look at what you are doing instead. You are buying cabbage, which costs two dollars and lasts a week. You are buying dried lentils, which cost pennies per serving. You are making your own probiotic ranch dressing using a carton of plain kefir that costs four dollars.

You have essentially eliminated a massive, recurring monthly bill.

This is not just about having more money in your checking account. This has a direct biological impact on your stomach.

Financial stress is one of the most common triggers for irritable bowel syndrome and chronic indigestion. When you are constantly worried about paying for expensive wellness products, or stressing over the cost of high-end organic health foods, your brain stays locked in a mild state of fight-or-flight.

Remember the vagus nerve? When you are stressed about money, the vagus nerve signals your digestive tract to slow down. The blood leaves your stomach. The motility halts.

By shifting your diet to cheap, reliable peasant foods—the oats, the beans, the root vegetables—you remove a massive source of daily anxiety. You know you can afford to eat this way for the rest of your life. You never have to worry about a subscription box of powders suddenly raising its prices.

The financial relief literally relaxes your nervous system, which in turn allows your stomach to digest your food in peace. The cheap food heals you twice—once through the fiber, and once through the peace of mind.

Handling the inevitable bad days

Now, here is the truth. Even with all this knowledge, even with a perfect grocery shopping routine, you are still going to have bad days.

You are a human being living in a chaotic world.

Someday, you are going to get a stomach bug. Someday, you are going to be so stressed at work that your digestion locks up for forty-eight hours. Someday, you will go on vacation, eat heavily processed food for five days straight, and come home feeling incredibly bloated and miserable.

When that happens, I want you to remember everything we have talked about.

Do not panic. Do not awfulize the situation and declare that your diet is a failure. Do not run to the internet looking for a new, magical supplement to bail you out.

You know exactly what to do.

If you are in acute pain from a flare-up, you immediately pivot to the 3-Day Gut Rest protocol. You boil some white rice. You bake a plain chicken breast. You heat up a mug of bone broth. You give your inflamed tissues the low-residue rest they desperately need.

If you are just sluggish and bloated from a bad weekend of eating, you do not need to rest the gut. You need to restart the engine. You drink a massive glass of water. You make the Kefir Overnight Oats. You take a walk to stimulate the migrating motor complex.

You do not need a doctor to fix a mild bad day, and you certainly do not need a wellness influencer. You just need to return to the basics.

The tools are already sitting in your kitchen.

The social power of sharing food

There is one last piece to this puzzle.

Throughout this book, we have focused heavily on the mechanics of your own body. We talked about your transit time, your fiber intake, and your specific bacterial strains. It is very easy to turn eating into a highly clinical, solitary, self-obsessed activity.

But food was never meant to be clinical.

For all of human history, eating has been a communal act. We gather around tables. We share large pots of stew. We break bread together.

When you isolate yourself because of your diet—when you cook a separate meal for yourself while your family eats something else, or when you refuse to go to dinner parties because you cannot control the ingredients—you lose the most important psychological benefit of eating. You lose connection.

When you sit at a table with people you care about, laughing and sharing a meal, your parasympathetic nervous system activates. This is the "rest and digest" mode. Your body floods with oxytocin. Your stomach muscles relax, your digestive enzymes flow freely, and your body optimally processes whatever you swallow.

A slightly imperfect meal eaten in a state of joy and connection will digest significantly better than a perfectly clean, high-fiber meal eaten alone in a state of high anxiety.

This is why we focused so heavily on making dinners that the whole family will actually eat. You have to bridge the gap. You have to bring your new habits to the communal table.

If you make the Hidden-Lentil Bolognese, do not eat it alone in the kitchen while your kids eat chicken nuggets. Serve it in a massive bowl in the center of the table. Let everyone dig in. Let them experience the comfort of the food, knowing quietly that you are feeding their microbiomes just as well as you are feeding your own.

Trusting your gut means trusting that you can participate in normal human life without breaking your body.

Your new baseline

Take a second to recognize how far you have come.

You used to think that the sour taste of fermented foods was impossible to overcome. Now, you know how to whisk white miso paste into your mashed potatoes for a massive hit of savory umami and live bacteria.

You used to think that eating healthy meant spending hours chopping raw vegetables for sad desk salads that left you exhausted by mid-afternoon. Now, you know how to build a heavy, complex grain bowl that keeps your blood sugar perfectly stable until dinner.

You used to think that a sudden bout of bloating meant you had an incurable medical condition. Now, you know it just means you need to chew your food better, drink more water, and give your gut a temporary rest.

You have removed the mystery from your digestion. It is no longer a black box that punishes you randomly. It is just an internal garden. You know how to water it, you know how to fertilize it, and you know how to leave it alone when it needs rest.

Final Action Step: Share the Table

Celebrate the changes you've made by sharing a nourishing meal with someone you care about.

1. Choose your favorite, most comforting recipe from this book—perhaps the **Mediterranean Chicken and Beans** or the **Gut-Friendly Tacos**.
2. Visit your local grocery store and buy the ingredients. Notice how simple, affordable whole foods can be compared with many products marketed as quick fixes.
3. Invite a friend, family member, or neighbor to join you for dinner.

4. Cook the meal and serve it with confidence. There is no need to apologize for it being “healthy”—it is simply delicious, satisfying food.
5. Sit down, enjoy the conversation, and share the meal. Notice how your body feels when you eat nourishing food in a relaxed setting with good company.

Final Takeaways

- Demanding absolute dietary perfection is an irrational trap; a robust, healthy microbiome easily handles occasional junk food or imperfect meals without suffering permanent damage.
- Letting go of the "patient identity" is crucial for long-term success; you are not fundamentally broken, you are simply learning to fuel a biological machine properly.
- The food matrix proves that isolated supplement pills cannot replicate the physical and chemical benefits of digesting whole, complex foods.
- Replacing expensive wellness products with cheap, ordinary staples like beans, oats, and cabbage actively reduces financial stress, which directly calms the nervous system and improves digestion.
- Eating in community activates the parasympathetic nervous system, proving that a relaxed, joyful meal digests far better than a perfect meal eaten in isolation and anxiety.

References

Bashiardes, S., Zilberman-Schapira, G., & Elinav, E. (2016). Use and exploitation of personalized diets in human microbiome research. American Journal of Gastroenterology, 111(7), 903–909.

Cardona, F., Andrés-Lacueva, C., Tulipani, S., Tinahones, F. J., & Queipo-Ortuño, M. I. (2013). Benefits of polyphenols on gut microbiota and implications in human health. Journal of Nutritional Biochemistry, 24(8), 1415–1422. https://doi.org/10.1016/j.jnutbio.2013.05.001

Deloose, E., Janssen, P., Depoortere, I., & Tack, J. (2012). The migrating motor complex: Control mechanisms and its role in health and disease. Nature Reviews Gastroenterology & Hepatology, 9(5), 271–285.

Dethlefsen, L., Huse, S., Sogin, M. L., & Relman, D. A. (2008). The pervasive effects of an antibiotic on the human gut microbiota, as revealed by deep 16S rRNA sequencing. PLoS Biology, 6(11), e280.

Furne, J. K., & Levitt, M. D. (1996). Factors influencing frequency of flatus emission by healthy subjects. Digestive Diseases and Sciences, 41(8), 1631–1635. https://doi.org/10.1007/BF02087912

Jacobs, D. R., & Tapsell, L. C. (2013). Food synergy: The key to a healthy diet. Proceedings of the Nutrition Society, 72(2), 200–206. https://doi.org/10.1017/S0029665112003011

Kim, M. H., & Kim, H. (2017). The roles of glutamine in the intestine and its implication in intestinal diseases. International Journal of Molecular Sciences, 18(5), 1051. https://doi.org/10.3390/ijms18051051

Lu, Q. Y., Summanen, P. H., Lee, R. P., Huang, J., Henning, S. M., Heber, D., Finegold, S. M., & Li, Z. (2019). Prebiotic potential and chemical composition of seven culinary spice extracts. Journal of Food Science, 84(8), 2092–2099.

Makki, K., Deehan, E. C., Walter, J., & Bäckhed, F. (2018). The impact of dietary fiber on gut microbiota in host health and disease. Cell Host & Microbe, 23(6), 705–715. https://doi.org/10.1016/j.chom.2018.05.012

Marco, M. L., Heeney, D., Binda, S., Cifelli, C. J., Cotter, P. D., Foligné, B., Gänzle, M., Kort, R., Pasin, G., Pihlanto, A., Smid, E. J., & Hutkins, R. (2017). Health benefits of fermented foods: Microbiota and beyond. Current Opinion in Biotechnology, 44, 94–102.

Marco, M. L., Sanders, M. E., Gänzle, M., Arrieta, M. C., Cotter, P. D., De Vuyst, L., Hill, C., Holzapfel, W., Lebeer, S., Merenstein, D., Reid, G., Wolfe, B. E., & Hutkins, R. (2021). The International Scientific Association for Probiotics and Prebiotics (ISAPP) consensus statement on fermented foods. Nature Reviews Gastroenterology & Hepatology, 18(3), 196–208.

McDonald, D., Hyde, E., Debelius, J. W., Morton, J. T., Gonzalez, A., Ackermann, G., … Knight, R. (2018). American Gut: An open platform for citizen science microbiome research. mSystems, 3(3), e00031-18. https://doi.org/10.1128/mSystems.00031-18

Sender, R., Fuchs, S., & Milo, R. (2016). Revised estimates for the number of human and bacteria cells in the body. PLOS Biology, 14(8), e1002533. https://doi.org/10.1371/journal.pbio.1002533

Slavin, J. (2013). Fiber and prebiotics: Mechanisms and health benefits. Nutrients, 5(4), 1417–1435. https://doi.org/10.3390/nu5041417

Smits, S. A., Leach, J., Sonnenburg, E. D., Gonzalez, C. G., Lichtman, J. S., Reid, G., … Sonnenburg, J. L. (2017). Seasonal cycling in the gut microbiome of the Hadza hunter-gatherers of Tanzania. Science, 357(6353), 802–806. https://doi.org/10.1126/science.aan4834

Su, G. L., Ko, C. W., Bercik, P., Falck-Ytter, Y., Sultan, S., Weizman, A. V., & Morgan, R. L. (2020). AGA clinical practice guidelines on the role of probiotics in the management of gastrointestinal disorders. Gastroenterology, 159(2), 697–705. https://doi.org/10.1053/j.gastro.2020.05.059

Tache, Y., Martinez, V., Million, M., & Wang, L. (2001). Stress and the gastrointestinal tract III. Stress-related alterations of gut motor function: Role of brain corticotropin-releasing factor receptors. American Journal of Physiology-Gastrointestinal and Liver Physiology, 280(2), G173–G177.

Thaiss, C. A., Zeevi, D., Levy, M., Zilberman-Schapira, G., Suez, J., Tengeler, A. C., Abramson, L., Katz, M. N., Korem, T., Zmora, N., Kuperman, Y., Biton, I., Gilad, S., Harmelin, A., Shapiro, H., Halpern, Z., Segal, E., & Elinav, E. (2014). Transkingdom control of microbiota diurnal oscillations promotes metabolic homeostasis. Cell, 159(3), 514–529.

Winter, C. K., & Katz, J. M. (2011). Dietary exposure to pesticide residues from commodities alleged to contain the highest contamination levels. Journal of Toxicology, 2011, Article 589674. https://doi.org/10.1155/2011/589674

Wu, G. D., Chen, J., Hoffmann, C., Bittinger, K., Chen, Y. Y., Keilbaugh, S. A., Bewtra, M., Knights, D., Walters, W. A., Knight, R., Sinha, R., Gilroy, E., Gupta, K., Baldassano, R., Nessel, L., Li, H., Bushman, F. D., & Lewis, J. D. (2011). Linking long-term dietary patterns with gut microbial enterotypes. Science, 334(6052), 105–108.

Yano, J. M., Yu, K., Donaldson, G. P., Shastri, G. G., Ann, P., Ma, L., … Hsiao, E. Y. (2015). Indigenous bacteria from the gut microbiota regulate host serotonin biosynthesis. Cell, 161(2), 264–276. https://doi.org/10.1016/j.cell.2015.02.047

Zeevi, D., Korem, T., Zmora, N., Israeli, D., Rothschild, D., Weinberger, A., Ben-Yacov, O., Lador, D., Avnit-Sagi, T., Lotan-Pompan, M., Suez, J., Mahdi, J. A., Matot, E., Malka, G., Kosower, N., Michal, P., Meirav, Z., Halpern, Z., Segal, E., & Elinav, E. (2015). Personalized nutrition by prediction of glycemic responses. Cell, 163(5), 1079–1094.

www.ingramcontent.com/pod-product-compliance
Lightning Source LLC
LaVergne TN
LVHW022107200926
848481LV00003B/1081
9798905991967